W0050698

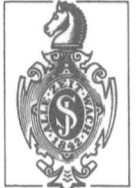

Thomas Sherwood A.K. Dixon
Desmond Hawkins M.L.J. Abercrombie

Roads to Radiology

An Imaging Guide to Medicine and Surgery

With 67 Figures

Springer-Verlag
Berlin Heidelberg New York 1983

M.L.J. Abercrombie, BSc, PhD.
Senior Research Associate, Department of Radiology,
University of Cambridge, UK

A.K. Dixon, MA, MB, MRCP, FRCR.
Lecturer in Radiology, University of Cambridge, UK

Desmond Hawkins, MA, MB, FRCP, FRCR.
Consultant Radiologist, Addenbrooke's Hospital, and
Clinical Dean, University of Cambridge, UK

Thomas Sherwood, MA, MB, FRCP, FRCR.
Professor of Radiology, University of Cambridge, UK

Library of Congress Cataloguing in Publication Data
Main entry under title: Roads to radiology.
Includes bibliographies and index. 1. Diagnosis, Radioscopic. I. Sherwood,
Thomas. [DNLM: 1. Radiography—Handbooks. 2. Radionuclide imaging—
Handbooks. WN 200 R628] RC78.R558   1982   616.07'572   82-16833
ISBN-13: 978-3-540-11801-5   e-ISBN-13: 978-1-4471-1341-6
DOI: 10.1007/ 978-1-4471-1341-6

The use of general descriptive names, trade marks, etc. in this publication,
even if the former are not to be taken as a sign that such names, as
understood by the Trade Marks and Merchandise Marks Act, may
accordingly be used freely by anyone.

This work is subject to copyright. All rights are reserved, whether the whole
or part of the material is concerned, specifically those of transflation,
reprinting, re-use of illustrations, broadcasting, reproduction by photo-
copying, machine or similar means, and storage in data banks. Under §54 of
the German Copyright Law where copies are made for other than private
use, a fee is payable to 'Verwertungsgesellschaft Wort', Munich.

© by Springer-Verlag Berlin Heidelberg 1983

Typeset by Photo-Graphics, Stockland, Honiton, Devon

2128/3916-543210

Preface

Our pocket-book has come about as a direct attempt to answer the needs of our clinical students. We have tried to use radiology as a magic window for looking at their patients' medical and surgical problems. The book is very simple and highly selective. A number of excellent introductory texts already exist for students seeking comprehensive and balanced accounts of radiology as a specialty. We have tried to keep close to our title: a good guide shows you a bare outline of where you might go, and makes sure you see the highlights. He will point to interesting places that deserve study, without going into them himself. Occasionally he may enlarge on a topic when the information is not readily available anywhere else (as in our chapter on the skull). And he will be ready to listen to students asking, perhaps rather shyly, some basic questions (as in our first and last chapters). We have taken Voltaire as our own guide: "Le secret d'ennuyer est ... de tout dire".

The book has been written by only a small group of all those teaching radiology at Cambridge. We wish to absolve our colleagues from all blame, and to thank them for generous support, especially in the loan of illustrations.

Cambridge, 1982   Thomas Sherwood

Contents

Acknowledgements

We thank Leonard Beard, MA, FIIP, FRPS, AIMBI, for painstaking work on the illustrations. Mary Watts did all our typing with aplomb and grace. We are also grateful to Drs C.D.R. Flower, A.H. Freeman, H. Holland, G.I. Verney and E.P. Wraight for advice and loan of illustrations. Jane Abercrombie is supported by the Nuffield Foundation. We thank our clinical students most of all: for commissioning and then criticizing the book — in short, for inspiration.

We are also grateful to Michael Jackson, Roger Dobbing, and many others at Springer-Verlag for producing the book.

1. Introduction: Medicine and Radiology

"Why do you want to be a doctor?" is a question often put across interview tables. Prospective medical students have almost certainly rehearsed an answer: "Because I am interested in people/human biology/life sciences" are some of the standard responses. "Because I want to care for sick people" is less popular—it sounds maudlin and somehow suspect. It may nevertheless be your real motive. It is in a long, honourable tradition, beginning in Western medicine with Hippocrates (floruit 420 BC). Note that Hippocrates himself pointed to pitfalls in the motive: the doctor as confidant of life or death is an extremely powerful figure, and that is a not unattractive post to most people. In his oath, which has come down to us by word of mouth, he is careful to warn against misuse of the massive trust patients place in their doctor: "In every house where I come I will enter only for the good of my patients, keeping myself far from all intentional ill-doing and all seduction .... All that may come to my knowledge in the exercise of my profession or outside my profession or in daily commerce with men, which ought not to be spread abroad, I will keep secret and will never reveal".

Doctors are privy to astounding confidences as a matter of course, for instance the news "I was playing with a vibrator, but then it disappeared" (Fig. 1.1).

This small book aims to guide medical students during their clinical studies in radiology. Radiology used to imply x-rays alone, but now covers the whole range of in vivo diagnostic imaging, including ultrasound, computed tomography (CT) and topographical nuclear medicine studies. An x-ray is a marvellous picture—hidden within it is often a detailed story allowing accurate diagnosis of what is wrong with a patient (Fig. 1.2).

The discovery of x-rays by Wilhelm Röntgen in 1895 might be taken as heralding the century of scientific medicine: at last, you might think, the business of diagnosis could be based on hard unbiased observation, not soft guesswork. This is not so—science at its best always begins with imagination, with a throw of ideas, followed by critical experiments to examine that hypothesis. Chapter 2 will take this view of science on into everyday medical practice, and Chap. 7 will examine problems of perception, of the statement "But it's true—I've seen it with my own eyes".

X-rays were welcomed with enthusiasm in the 1890s. The news about the magic new rays spread like wildfire. Röntgen's chance discovery was debated in London in January 1896, a month after its publication. Soon

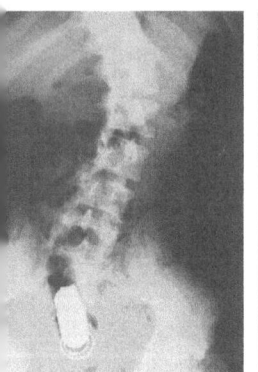

Fig. 1.1. ▲

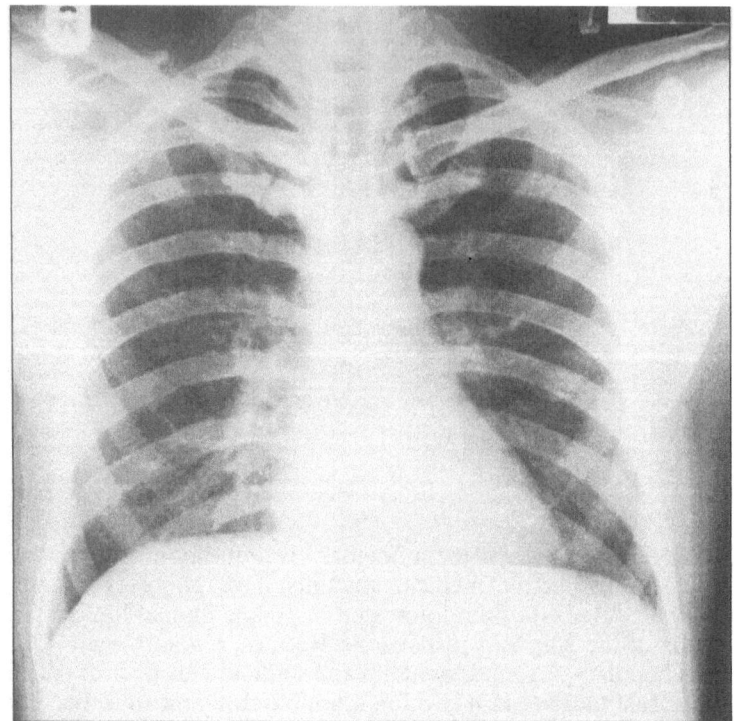

Fig. 1.2a. ▲

Fig. 1.2b. ▼

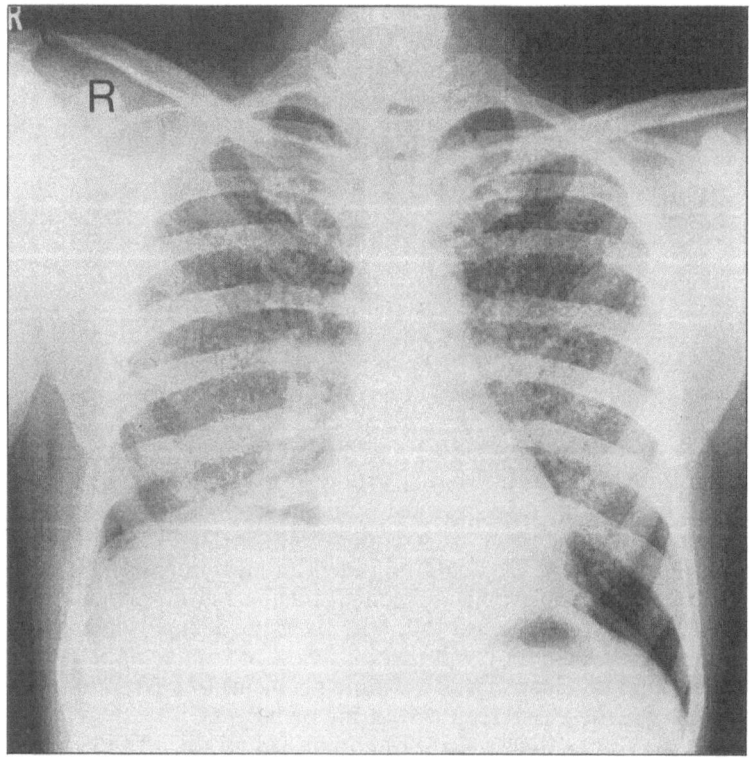

2

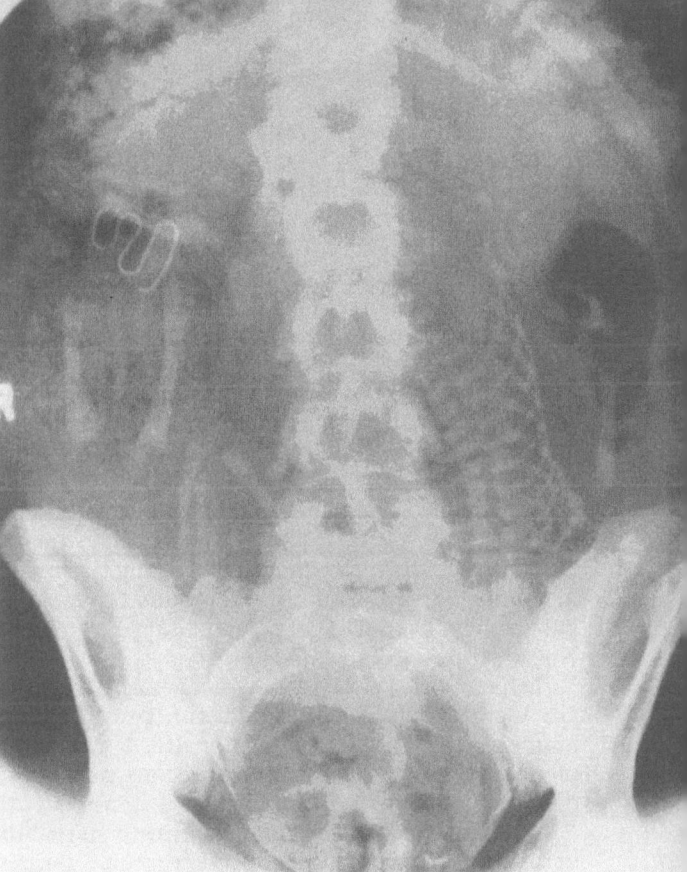

Fig. 1.3. There are two people on this radiograph, but such films are now rare because ultrasound is a better way of looking at the fetus. Note two dense (*white*) man-made objects—the lead letter outside the mother's abdomen, and the rather ineffective intra-uterine contraceptive device within it. Mother and baby are well, but there is an unusual finding on this film: the layer of sclerosis (*white*) in each ilium next to the sacroiliac joints. This is sometimes seen in pregnancy as a response to strain at this joint, and remains as a lifelong but quite unimportant abnormality.

everyone was carrying out x-ray examinations. Fractures could be diagnosed with certainty, because bone with its high calcium content showed a clear outline, separate from surrounding soft tissues. It was soon found that there were three basic photographic densities to juggle with on radiographs (Fig. 1.3):

White — the bones.
Black — gas in the lungs and the bowel, and also fat.
Grey — all other tissues (muscle, blood etc.), the "soft tissues".

Fig. 1.1. Vibrator up rectum. You may think this picture in poor taste, but the problems behind it are real. Note that the patient has a scoliosis, and that the plastic upper part of the device is shown clearly as a radiolucent (*black*) structure. Fat is a naturally occurring substance of low atomic number that will appear similarly black on radiographs.

Fig. 1.2.a Normal chest x-ray in a young man. **b** A month later he is very sick, and both lungs are studded with tiny tubercles, about the size of a millet seed. He has developed blood-borne, miliary tuberculosis.

Experiments to make other organs visible by filling them with radio-opaque substances before x-raying were quickly under way. The first arteriograms were done at the turn of the century by instilling red lead into the arterial system of cadavers. Barium sulphate, a non-absorbable and therefore safe substance in the gut, could be given to patients to drink: it made their whole intestinal tract visible. Substances like lead, barium and iodine are radio-opaque because they have a high atomic number: their atoms are good at stopping (absorbing) x-rays.

By the 1920s radiologists were setting up as specialist physicians to deal with the new techniques. In the same decade an unknown young medical registrar in Berlin had the idea of passing a catheter into an arm vein, and on up the venous system into the right side of the heart. He carried this out on himself, and then walked to the x-ray department. The spirits of the accompanying young colleague who was to fluoroscope him gave out at this stage, and he left in fright. Forssmann had to fluoroscope himself, using a mirror to see the x-ray image of the catheter bouncing about in his heart: the first cardiac catheterizaton. Forssmann repeated the experiments on himself but was laughed out of court, and disappeared into the country. He received a Nobel prize, but 25 years later.

Radiographs are static x-ray images, produced on photographic film. They are the standard stock-in-trade of x-ray departments, and are taken by *radiographers,* skilled professionals. A radiograph is thus a split-second record. Care is necessary in reconstructing real-time events in four-dimensional patients from this two-dimensional "frozen" image (Fig. 1.4).

A patient can also be examined directly in real time by a continuous stream of x-rays, and his living image viewed on a fluorescent or television screen. Such *fluoroscopy,* or *screening*, is generally carried out by *radiologists*, who are diagnostic physicians.

Figure 1.4 shows the use of parenteral contrast media, opacifying internal organs by their selective excretion (kidneys, gall-bladder) or by direct injection (arteries, veins). In this way the first intravenous urograms (IVU) for in vivo opacification of the urinary tract were also done in the 1920s. The early steps along the major avenues of medical x-ray technique were all taken in the first 40 years after Röntgen's discovery. A 1930's IVU is not all that different from today's examination (Fig. 1.5). By the 1950s, nuclear medicine studies were under way: functional maps of organs marked out by radioactive isotope labels (see Chap. 3). Radar was a success story of World War II, but did not make its mark in medicine till the 1960s. Ultrasound scans are structural, sectional maps of the body, determined not by the atomic number of the tissues, as in x-rays, but by their acoustic elasticity (see Chap. 5). Diagnostic ultrasound is harmless, a unique advantage by comparison with x-ray and nuclear medicine techniques.

Computed tomography (CT) is a 1970's development. It results in superbly detailed cross-sectional maps of the body, using a pencil x-ray beam which traverses the organism, a scintillation counter (not photographic film!) as sensor on the other side, and a computer to reconstruct images (see Chap. 4). The technique has wrought a revolution in the practice of neurology and neurosurgery. Its impact on medical practice in other areas will probably be less startling, but nevertheless far reaching.

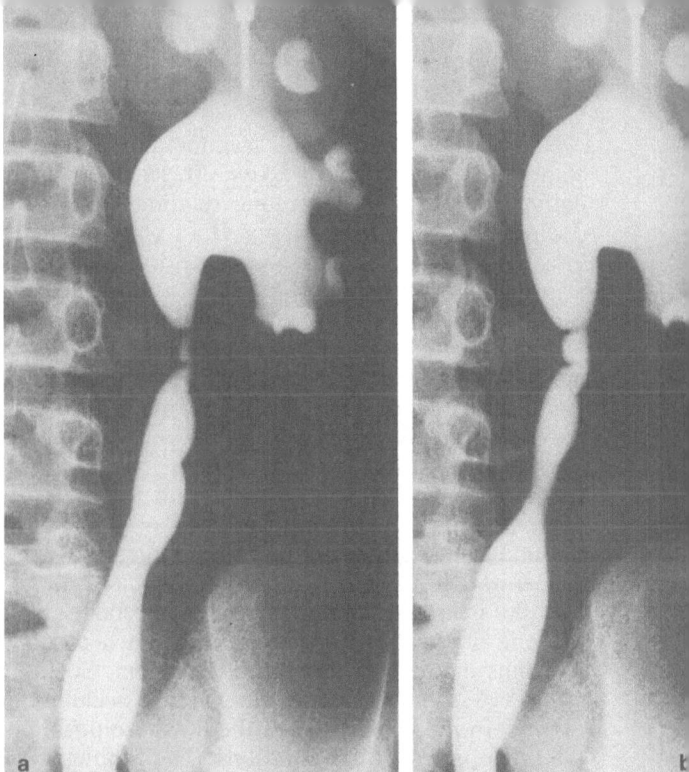

Fig. 1.4.a and **b** Two views of a pelviureteric junction during an antegrade pyelogram—percutaneous puncture of a renal pelvis to test for obstruction. Peristaltic waves are seen travelling down the ureter.

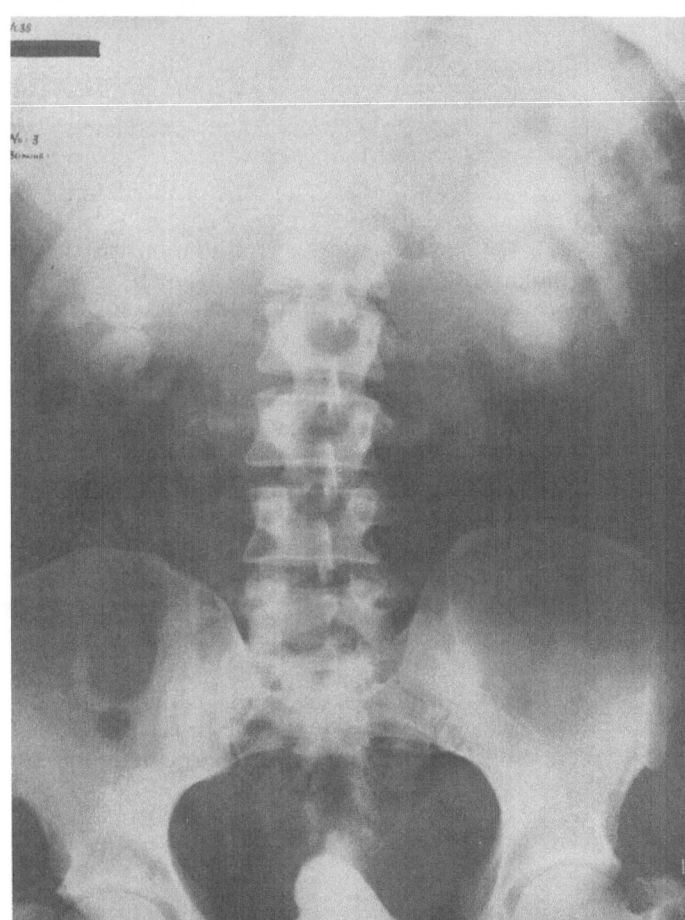

Fig. 1.5. An IVU dated 1938. Contrast medium excreted by the kidneys outlines considerably dilated calices on both sides. The cause is a large bladder stone—the very dense (*white*) object at the bottom of the film.

Radiologists wielding CT scanners illustrate some interesting problems of contemporary medicine. Even 20 years after Röntgen's discovery, most patients stood in a one-to-one relationship with their doctor: he was *their* doctor, they were *his* patients. If an x-ray was needed, he would "order" it, look at it, and decide what was to be done as a result. The suffering individual was his only concern, and he was trusted to leave no stone unturned in that cause.

The basic tenet of personal care for the sick individual rightly remains a maxim of medical teaching, but it has inevitably become overlaid with the complexities of the age. Teams of medical and paramedical personnel are now often involved in a patient's care, with smudged lines of responsibility. Experts and tests abound: patients are "worked-up" for diagnosis and treatment (see Chap. 2). Leaving no stone unturned can be an extremely distressing experience for a patient, as well as a costly exercise for society. We cannot be endlessly generous and yet fair: if we spend all our resources on one desperately ill patient with a hopeless disease, we shall not be able to cope with the next two, who may have correctable disorders.

Medical students will recognize a much older conflict here: between the demands of the individual and of society. Society may argue that it cannot afford CT scanners, and the individual can claim that he is not having the best of modern medicine without them. These problems are sketched here to set the scene, not to offer solutions. The following are guide-ropes as students move through the maze in radiology.

1) "I will prescribe regimen for the good of my patient according to my ability and my judgement and never do harm to anyone" (Hippocrates). The need for sensible judgement has been an accepted part of good medical practice for over 2000 years, and it is too late to be afraid of it now. How can we learn to be good judges?

2) Patients posing a diagnostic problem fare best where radiologists act as clinicians' consultants. An x-ray request is then not a demand for a piece of irradiated film, but for a consultation on the diagnostic problem. Using radiology departments simply as medical photography or data delivery machines, spewing out x-ray films like a sausage factory, is unkind and bad for patients, depressingly uncritical for doctors, and no good at all for the hospital purse. Note that the choice of words will help to get this right for the newcomer: an x-ray is not "ordered" (like dinner) but "requested" (like any other consultation between professionals). If unsure what to ask for next, discuss the problem with the radiologist.

3) Radiology departments are one of the most expensive items in any hospital budget. The radiologists running them may well be dedicated doctors with a Hippocratic devotion to the needs of the individual. But because they have to provide for the next patient 5 minutes on, they will inevitably be very conscious of society's needs also. "Is this really worth doing?" may be asked by them not because they are idle, or do not care, but because they are busy and care very much.

4) Medical students entering a clinical school are once more in a position they have experienced several times: the lowest rung of a new ladder. Radiology departments can be particularly intimidating places because they

are full of impenetrable gadgets, and of experts doing complex things. The feeling easily arises that this is all too much for the newcomer, and that he will only make an ignorant nuisance of himself if he ventures a foot or a question. This is a pity: by and large radiologists are jacks-of-all-clinical-trades who enjoy contacts outside their specialty, and are ready to talk and explain. As a student I was taught "follow your patients into the post-mortem room"; the contemporary extension of that must be "follow your patients into the radiology department". You will be welcome.

2. Diagnosis

"The most important difference between a good and indifferent clinician lies in the amount of attention paid to the story of a patient" (Farquhar Buzzard 1933). A contemporary study supports this aphorism. Sandler (1979) found that the history decided 56% of all diagnoses (and 46% of all management) in his medical outpatients. Clinical examination accounted for 17% of diagnostic decisions, and investigations for only 23%. This does not add up to 100%—the hallmark of an honest study—because no diagnosis could be made in 4% of patients.

The process of diagnosis is obviously a subtle interplay of many trains of thought and observation. This begins the moment a patient enters a doctor's field of vision—perhaps even before that if there is a referral letter to be read. Great physicians have stressed the importance of beginning with the first look: how the patient enters the room, sits down, opens his story. A history emerges, and the good clinician listens and looks, interjects a key question here, gently jogs the patient on there. All the while, diagnostic ideas are turning over in his mind: "This man says he's tired and has slowed up no end just recently—he looks a bit leaden—could he have myxoedema? No, his skin was warm and sweaty when we shook hands just now, so that's wrong. How about anaemia and its causes..."

Note that the human computer does here, quite unstoppably, what it is good at: continuously weighing up complex choices around a small number of hypotheses, probably at most two or three at a time. It examines the multiple facets of these few guesses, tosses them around, rejects the unlikely hypothesis, and moves on to the next likely idea. Note also that a real computer would act differently: as an information store, displaying at once a hundred possible diagnoses for a particular symptom.

At the end of the history, the skilled clinician will either be on to *the* diagnosis, or know the two or three most likely contenders. If he is experienced, he uses the clinical examination as a brief survey tool sweeping across the whole scene, then focussing onto his guesses in order to confirm or refute them. If he is an inexperienced medical student, he will have to do a meticulous A–Z examination, checking on everything because the best diagnostic ideas may not yet have occurred to him.

The process of investigations is at best an extension of the clinical method. An x-ray examination is a way of checking on a hypothesis: does this patient indeed have old pulmonary tuberculosis ("chest x-ray please"), and now anaemia because of a colonic carcinoma ("barium enema please")? If he does not, we will have to go on to the next most likely idea, and examine that.

This is a step-by-step, trial-and-error path into the challenge of making a diagnosis. It fits in well with the way the human brain works, but you may say that it has nothing to do with science. Is it not the triumph of scientific medicine to have moved away from everything smacking of mere guesswork? Does not scientific method demand unbiased observation of the facts? Surely the doctor should start by gathering in the evidence of the history and the clinical examination, then add to it the weight of facts derived from multiple investigations. The more data the better: at the end of the process we shall review the evidence impartially, and the diagnosis will pop out. If it does not, we have not worked hard enough at data collecting.

The expression "diagnostic work-up" sums up this approach. It is unkind for the patient, who is subjected to too many tests, uncritical for the doctor, who ticks an investigation list, and it is very costly. That the diagnostic work-up is also deeply unscientific is perhaps the most telling indictment. Scientific method can be seen to work by just the trial-and-error steps described for the patient–physician encounter. Scientists begin with a spark, an idea ("I wonder if that would explain it"), and go on to experiments which test the hypothesis. If they are great scientists, the experiments will be breathtakingly sharp, direct and elegant.

This view of science has been put eloquently by Popper (see Magee 1973), Medawar (1969) and Campbell (1976). These sources are well worth reading if you need support against the onslaught of the many textbooks or lecturers who champion the information-gathering, innocent-eye approach to science. The scientist's mind is no more a clean slate, to be filled with unbiased primary observations, than any other man's.

That the claims of scientific method, humanity, economy and perception should all come together here to pull in the same direction, away from the diagnostic work-up, may seem too cunning a piece of good luck. Disprove it!

There are important consequences to this view of diagnostic affairs in radiology (Sherwood 1978). They should influence how you look at an x-ray or other diagnostic image, and how you investigate your patients.

Looking at an x-ray

It will be very hard to extract a story from the film if you have no notion what kind of things you are looking for. Radiologists do quite often make chance observations on films, and sometimes these bear on the clinical problem. That is a hit-or-miss process, because the inner eye is not good at sweeping a field containing hundreds of equally weighted information bits. But if you have a young patient with sudden one-sided chest pain and suspect a pneumothorax, you will have every chance of making the difficult key observation: the tiny hairline edge of a lung that has moved away from the chest wall (Fig. 2.1). You and all radiologists need good clinical information when looking at an x-ray film, in order to tell the best possible story about what is really going on.

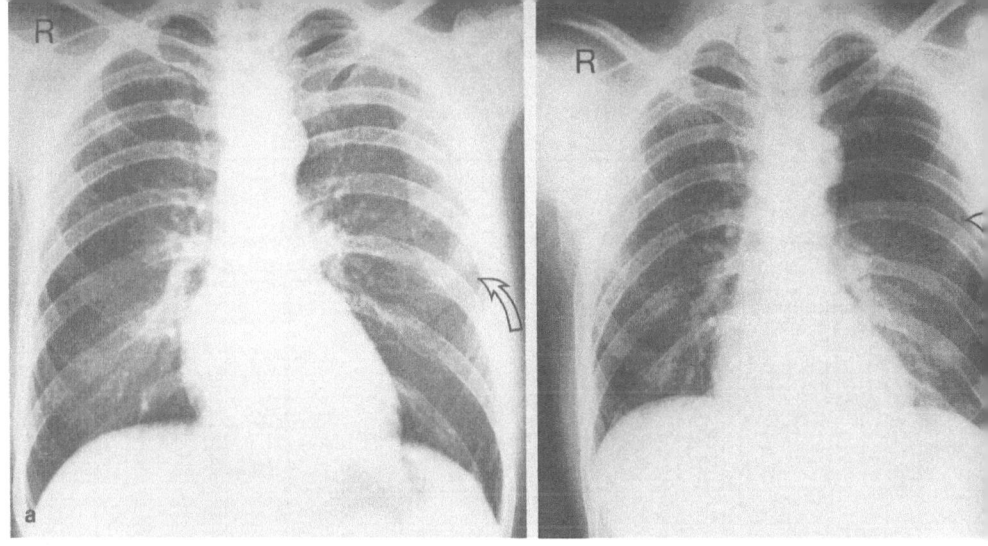

Fig. 2.1.a A patient with a spontaneous left pneumothorax—the lung edge is difficult to see on this standard inspiration film (*arrow*). **b** Diagnosis is a little easier on this expiration film (*arrows*). Note that there are no lung markings in the air-filled pleural space distal to the lung.

It can be shown that biased observers, ready to generate good hypotheses from the clinical background, perform better than "blind" readers of radiographs—a nice paradox which should no longer come as a surprise.

Diagnostic pathways

Good doctors, like good scientists, choose elegantly simple and direct experiments for checking on their ideas. Building step by step on the next likely diagnosis often means building critical diagnostic pathways through a maze of possible investigations. It is a particular problem that most tests in medicine do not provide black/white, yes/no answers. A patient with a renal mass seen on the IVU should have an ultrasound scan next, to see if the lesion is fluid or solid. If fluid, the mass is probably a simple cyst, and of no further importance. But there is a perhaps 5% chance that the ultrasound scan is wrong, and that an unusual renal tumour may be present. We therefore spread a safety net below the patient, in order not to let him drop into diagnostic limbo just because one test has produced a false negative result about an important diagnostic possibility.

A simple diagnostic pathway for the renal mass problem is shown in Fig. 2.2. Here we say we will puncture all renal cysts thought to be doubtful on ultrasound evidence, in order to carry us across the 5% error rate. Renal puncture is a simple outpatient procedure, done under local anaesthesia (Fig. 2.3). Occasionally we will then puncture a renal tumour. Follow-up studies have shown that this does not impair the patient's chances, and we will of course know at once from the puncture findings that all is not well (Fig. 2.4).

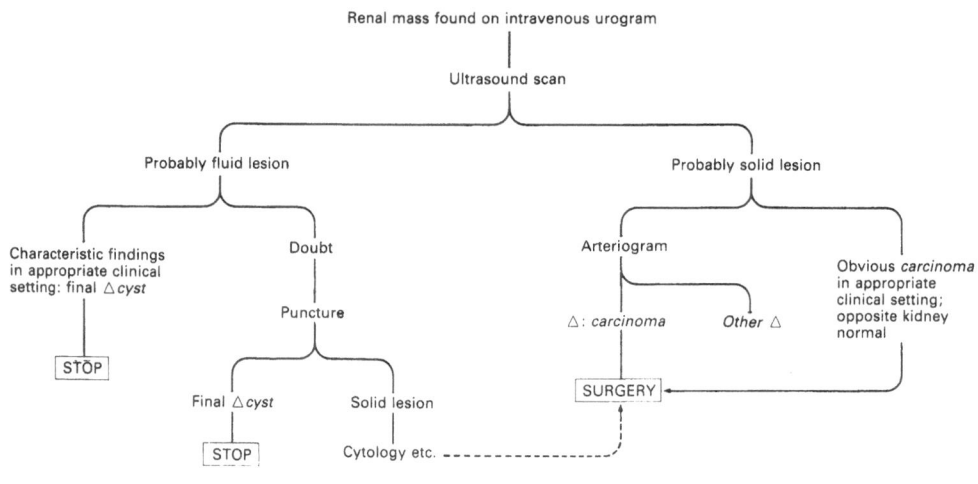

Fig. 2.2. Old diagnostic pathway for renal mass.

Fig. 2.3.a On this IVU there is a circular avascular (*black*) lesion in the left upper renal pole (*arrow*), about the size of a penny. **b** Percutaneous puncture of the renal cyst, replacing its contents with contrast medium.

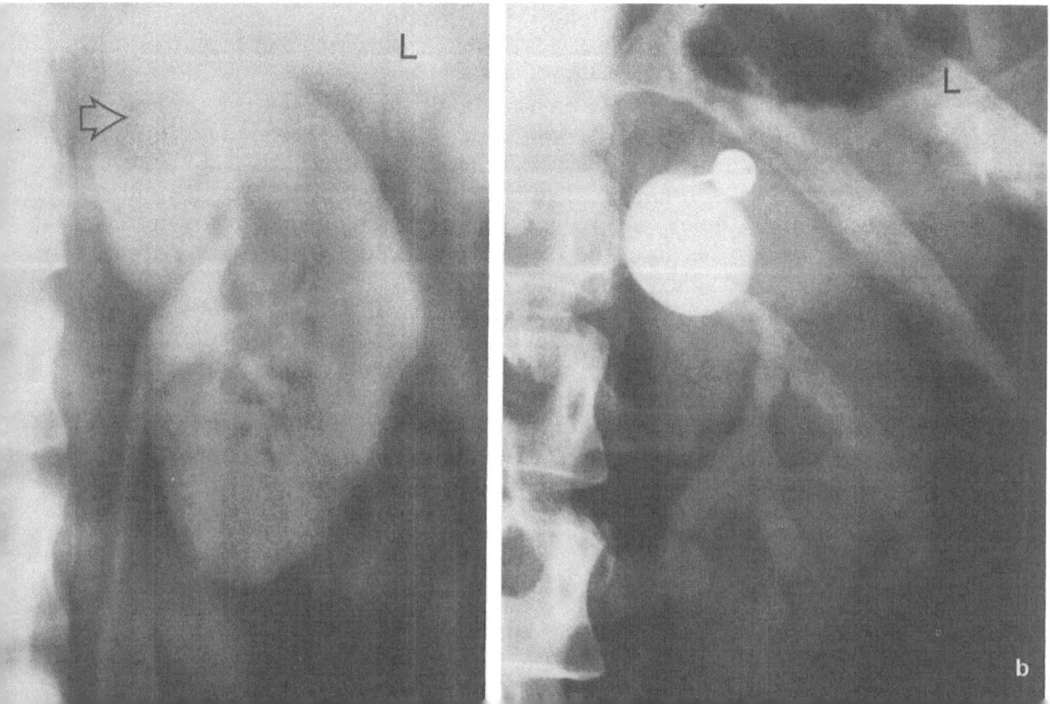

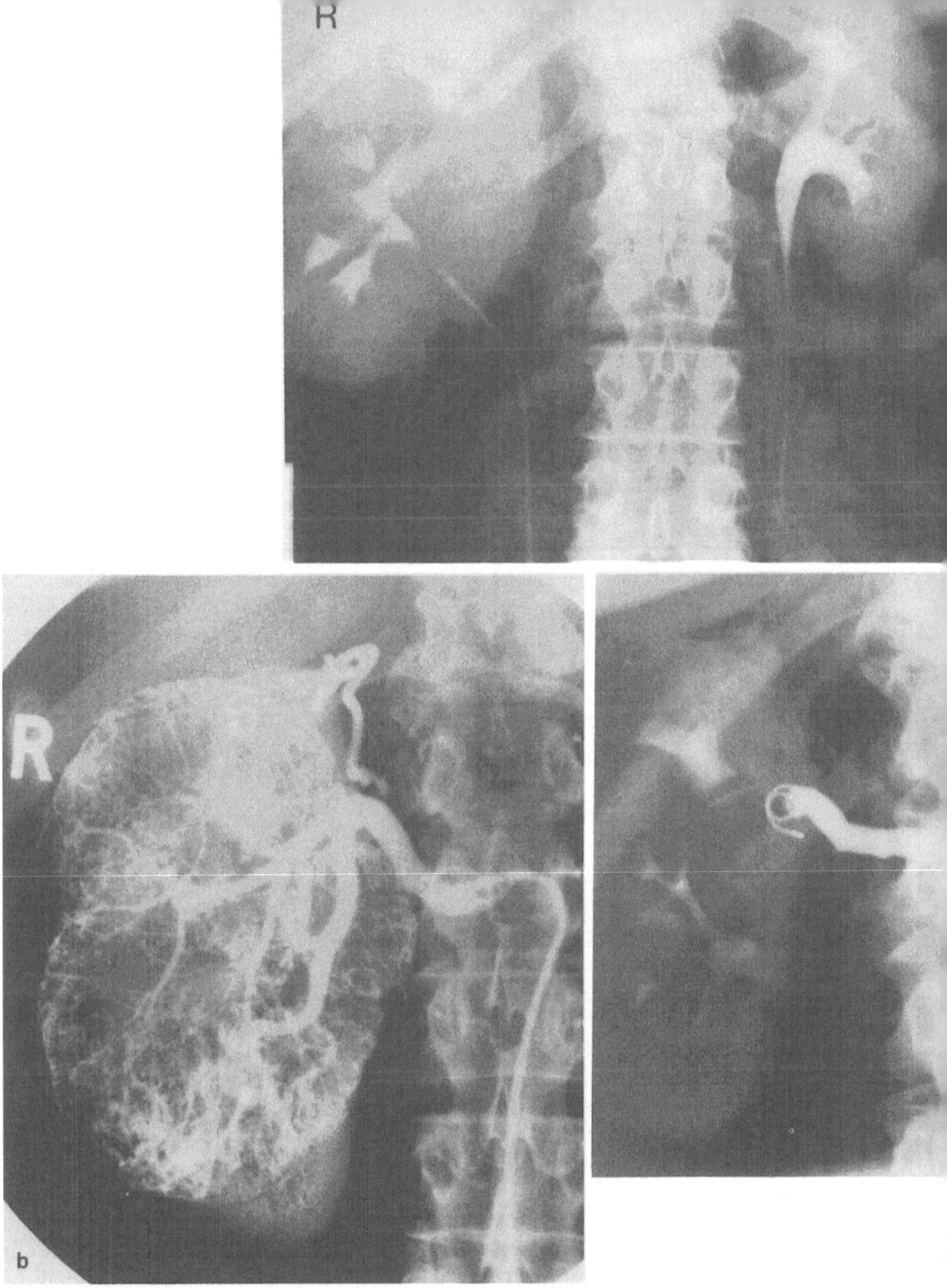

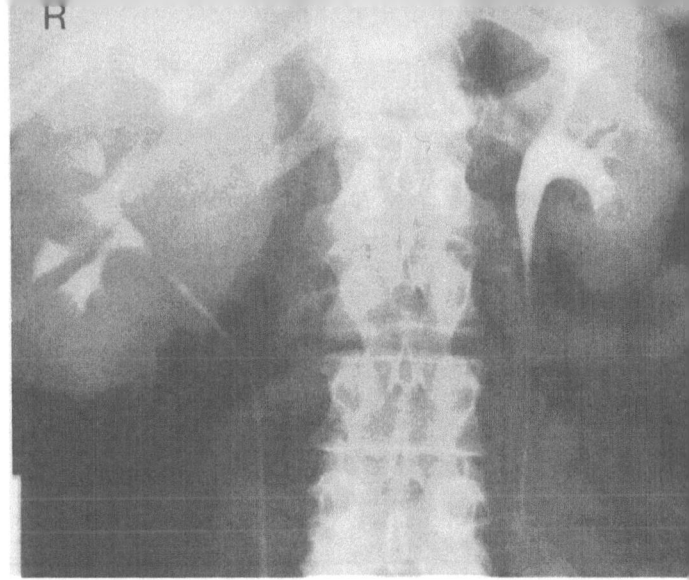

Fig. 2.4.a The right kidney appears misshapen on this IVU by comparison with the left. **b** A catheter has been put into the right renal artery, and the selective arteriogram obtained in this way shows a very large mass within this kidney. Only the tip of the lower renal pole remains normal—the abnormal arterial pattern within the mass makes renal carcinoma the likely diagnosis. **c** At the end of the arteriogram a small wire coil has been injected through the catheter in order to occlude the renal artery. This manoeuvre makes for easier surgery of such large, vascular tumours.

13

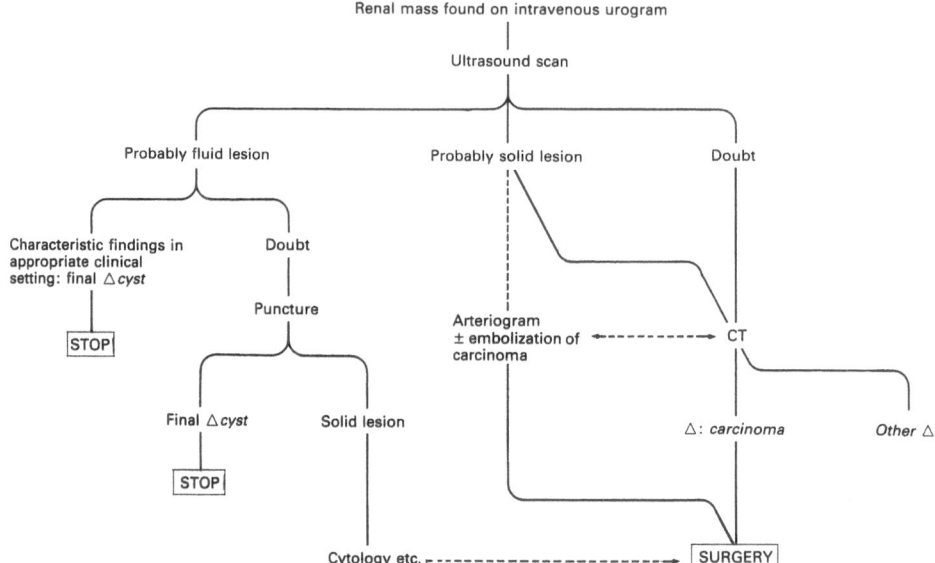

Fig. 2.5. New diagnostic pathway for renal mass.

Clinical judgement has an immediate impact on each step of a diagnostic pathway. The patient may be elderly, and the renal mass a chance finding on an IVU done for other reasons, say bladder outflow obstruction. On wholly characteristic IVU and ultrasound findings of a renal cyst, we may very properly decide that the small chance of missing an unlikely renal carcinoma is not important to this patient's life chances. It is in his best interests to stop the diagnostic pathway in its tracks there and then, without renal puncture.

The advent of CT scanning is changing ideas about how to tackle the investigation of a renal mass. At present a diagnostic pathway on this topic might look as in Fig. 2.5. Because of new techniques and new knowledge we will always wish to have open minds about changing tack on diagnostic problems. The whole approach implies close co-operation between clinician and investigators, ready to discuss the particular features of an individual patient. In a hospital this works particularly well in the setting of regular weekly clinico-radiological conferences.

Sensitivity and specificity of tests

Blood clots lodging in pulmonary arteries, having been swept up from thrombi in leg veins, often make up a difficult diagnosis. Clinical findings can be indeterminate, and the chest x-ray is usually unhelpful. A radionuclide lung scan is the next sensible step. Radioactively labelled microspheres are injected intravenously, and thus into the pulmonary arterial bed. Their numbers are too small to cause any flow impairment, but via a gamma camera they provide a functional map of regional lung perfusion. If the perfusion scan is normal (Fig. 2.6), the probability of pulmonary emboli is extremely low. The test has great *sensitivity:* it picks up all perfusion abnormalities, and a false negative result is highly unlikely. On the other hand, if the scan is abnormal and shows perfusion defects (Fig. 2.7), the patient may have pulmonary emboli, or pneumonia, or emphysema, or... . The test's *specificity* is low: something is certainly amiss with lung perfusion in this patient, but this may be a false positive result as regards the diagnosis of pulmonary emboli. The abnormal perfusion scan can be made much more specific by following it up at once with a radionuclide ventilation scan. Lung segments harbouring pulmonary emboli show a characteristic mismatch between impaired perfusion and normal ventilation.

The sensitivity and specificity of diagnostic tests are important for designing sensible diagnostic pathways. The current use of these terms is not always in keeping with what you might expect (McNeil et al. 1975). Remember that a highly sensitive test is good at picking out the patients who *do* have the disease under suspicion (few false negatives), a highly specific one those who do *not* have this particular disease (few false positives).

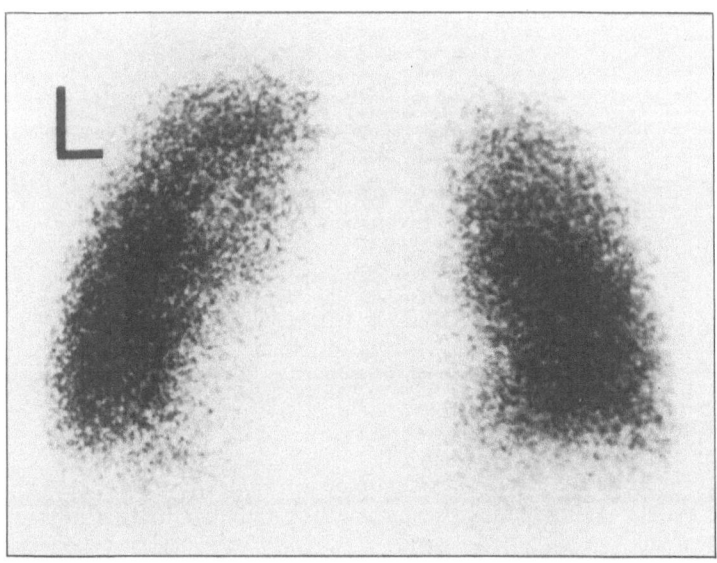

Fig. 2.6. Normal lung perfusion scan (posterior view, i.e. seen from behind). ^{99m}Tc microspheres have been injected intravenously, and carried to the pulmonary capillary bed. The radioactivity (*black*) marks out an even perfusion picture.

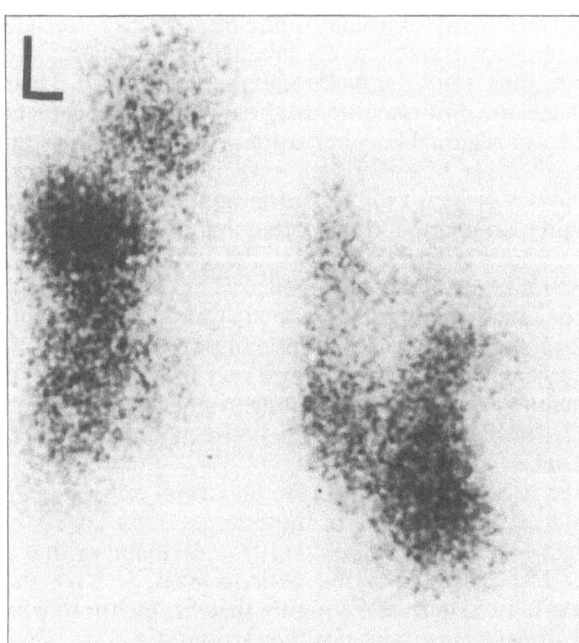

◀ Fig. 2.7.a

▼ Fig. 2.7.b

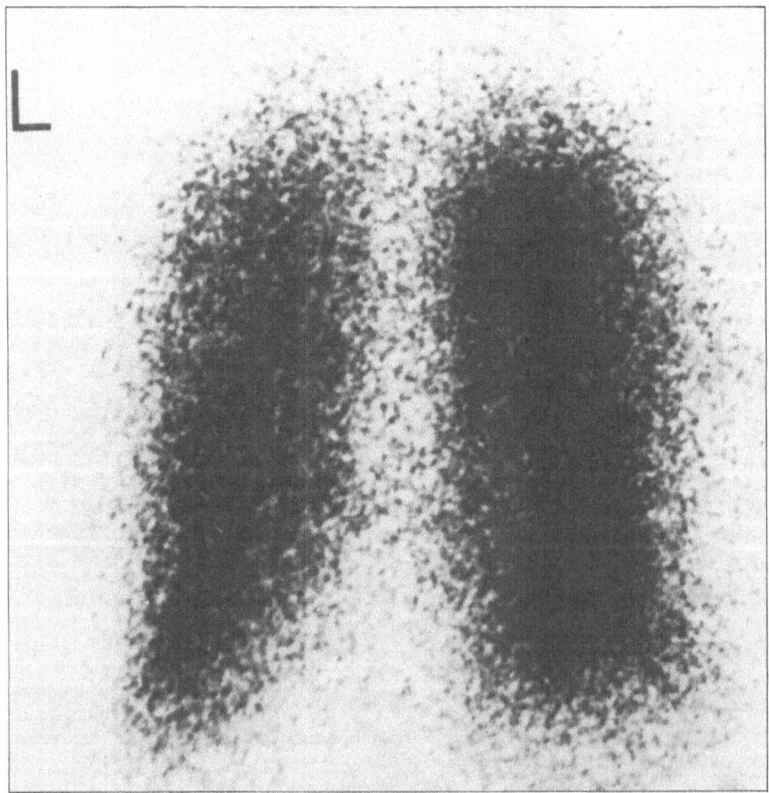

Fig. 2.7.a Perfusion scan in a patient with multiple pulmonary emboli. Note the very many defects in the black perfusion map of both lungs. **b** The same patient has taken a breath of ^{133}Xe gas, showing a normal ventilation map. A mismatch between impaired perfusion and normal ventilation is a characteristic diagnostic picture in pulmonary embolism.

◄—————————————————————————————————

Conclusion

Proper diagnosis tends to be put on a pedestal in clinical medicine, but it is, of course, only a means to an end: proper management of the patient. Note that this includes prognosis. If we can reach an accurate diagnosis of even a hopeless disease by a good, quick route, the patient can be spared further diagnostic agonies, and he or his relatives kindly prepared for the likely outcome. CT scanning in pancreatic carcinoma is a good example. On the other hand, some diagnoses are not worth pursuing. About 10% of the adult population suffer from hypertension. In the adult with a raised blood pressure but normal renal function and normal urine examination, a possible underlying renal cause like renal artery stenosis will not affect initial management (drug treatment). It is therefore pointless, unkind and wasteful to do routine renograms or IVUs here.

It would be idle to pretend that the ideas in this chapter are generally accepted, or that they are easy to apply in practice across the whole field of medical endeavour. The topics of renal masses and pulmonary emboli are two of the very few where they have been tested (jaundice and intracerebral haemorrhage are other examples). A very great deal remains to be done if we are to extend these ways of kind, scientific and economic diagnosis. We need more, not less, science to get this right—a challenge to encourage you and me into behaving like scientists in everyday clinical medicine.

References

Buzzard F (1933) Preparation for medical practice. Lancet ii:820 (This one page of advice for the medical student is well worth reading.)

Campbell EJM (1976) Basic science, science and medical education. Lancet i:134–136

McNeil BJ, Keeler E, Adelstein SJ (1975) Primer on certain elements of medical decision making. N Engl J Med 293:211–215

Magee B (1973) Popper. Fontana/Collins, London (The easiest way into Popper's work and thought is via this short study in the Fontana Modern Masters series.)

Medawar PB (1969) Induction and intuition in scientific thought. Methuen, London

Sandler G (1979) Costs of unnecessary tests. Br Med J ii:21–24

Sherwood T (1978) Science in radiology. Lancet i:594–595

3. Bones

Fractures

Breaks in bones can be quite obvious (Fig. 3.1). Sometimes diagnosis is difficult (Fig. 3.2). It is very important to get this right: the injured are generally fit people who can be restored to a normal existence provided the hurt is correctly diagnosed and treated. In this respect trauma and accident work is vitally different from the medicine and surgery concerned with temporary comforting and salvage of mortally sick patients. The preventable errors strike the harder: not recognizing a disabling elbow fracture in a child (Fig. 3.3) makes up a tragedy.

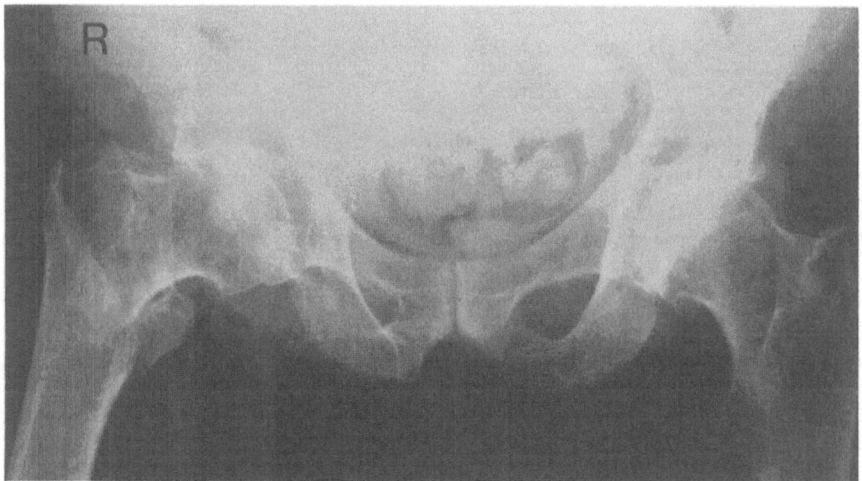

Fig. 3.1. An obvious fracture of the right femoral neck.

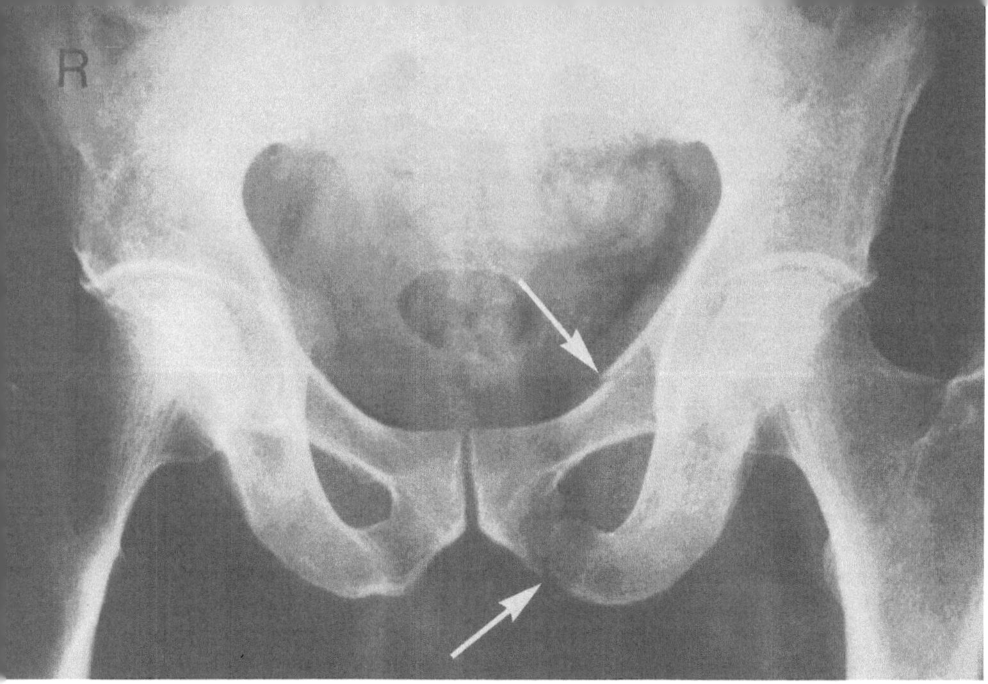

Fig. 3.2. ▲   Fig. 3.3.a ▼   Fig. 3.3.l

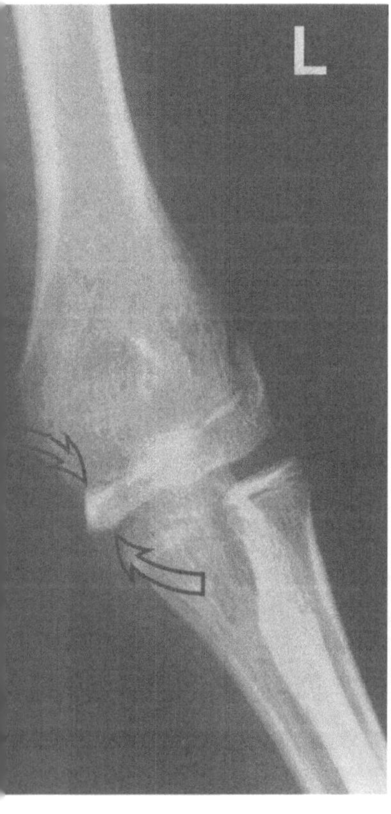

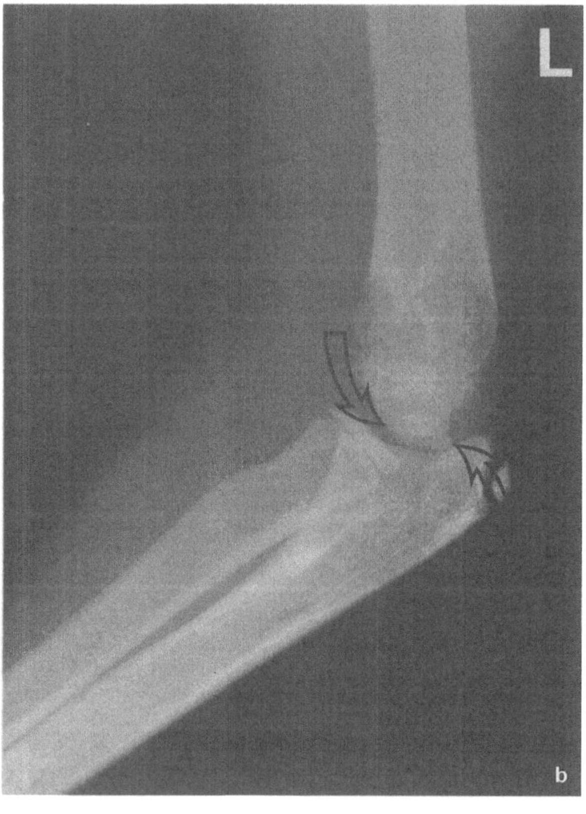

Fig. 3.2. This patient also has fractures following a fall, but they are a little more difficult than that shown in Fig. 3.1. *Arrows* point to the breaks in the pelvic bone. The clues here are the steps in the outline of the rings making up the pelvic inlet and obturator foramen.

◀————————————————

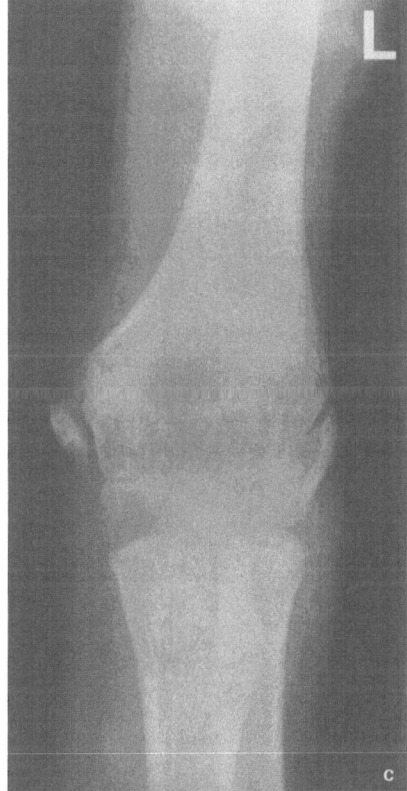

Fig. 3.3.a and **b** This boy has fallen on his arm, and his elbow is now swollen and very tender. The *arrows* point to the lesion. **c** A later film after correction, to show what this elbow should look like. The earlier films show an avulsed and badly misplaced medial epicondyle epiphysis.

First principles

1) *Two radiographs* at right angles to each other ("AP and lateral") are usually needed for examining a suspect bone. The names of the projections describe the path of the x-ray beam through the part.

Exceptions: (a) An oblique rather than lateral view is sometimes appropriate as the second projection, for instance for the foot. (b) A single AP film suffices for a few bones, e.g. the pelvis. Even here, if a fracture of the hip is suspected, a special lateral view must be done. Do not hesitate to ask radiographers or radiologists for advice if you are in doubt over anything.

2) *Deformity and discontinuity* of bone are the obvious hallmarks of fractures. These may need very careful tracing of bony outlines on the radiograph to be sure all is well.

3) *Joint effusions* are a helpful pointer to a fracture nearby. The elbow is the best example, because an effusion here almost always means a fracture,

21

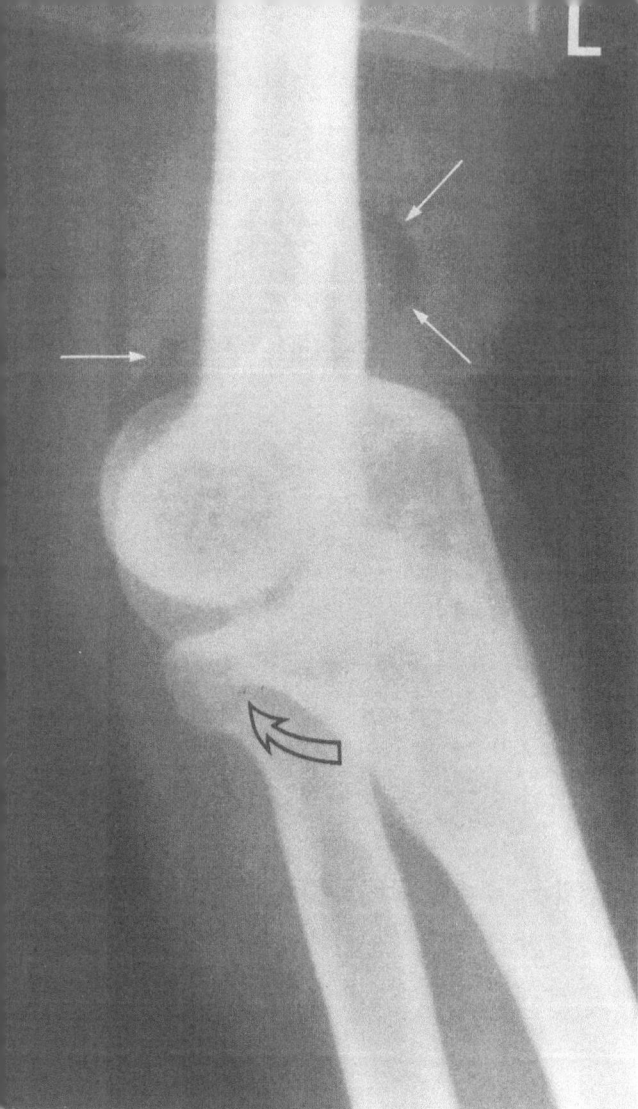

Fig. 3.4. Elbow joint effusion—
note displacement of anterior and
posterior fat pads (*small arrows*).
The *large curved arrow* points to
the radial head fracture.

but the bony defect can be difficult to make out. Fat pads outlining the joint capsule are radiolucent, and their displacement indicates an effusion (Fig. 3.4).

Rule of thumb: if a posterior fat pad is seen at all in the elbow, an effusion with a likely fracture is present.

4) *Follow-up films* are always worth while if in doubt. This is because bone is resorbed along a fracture line, so that an obvious radiolucent break is seen here 10 days or so after the insult. Should you be unsure whether a fracture is present, treat the patient as if it is (i.e. rest or immobilize the part), and re-x-ray.

5) *Children:* fractures here are different because the lines of weakness and the elasticity of a growing bone are not the same as in adults. Two particular

difficulties arise. (a) *Epiphyseal injuries.* Displacement of epiphyses rather than bony breaks occurs quite readily as the first injury when a child's bone comes under stress (see Fig. 3.3). Knowing the correct place and development of epiphyses is therefore important for orthopaedic surgeons and radiologists. The hallowed way of dealing with this problem by the inexperienced in the middle of the night is to x-ray the corresponding contralateral healthy part for comparison. This means unnecessary radiation to the patient, is often not as helpful as might be hoped, and is altogether overdone. In an Accident and Emergency department you should have access to either an immediate expert radiological consultation or, second best, to a standard atlas of bone development. X-raying the opposite side of the body is third best. (b) *Greenstick fractures.* Children's bones may just crumple under trauma, their elasticity preventing a clean break. The most common example is the lower end of the radius; you will certainly need a lateral view here to see this properly (Fig. 3.5).

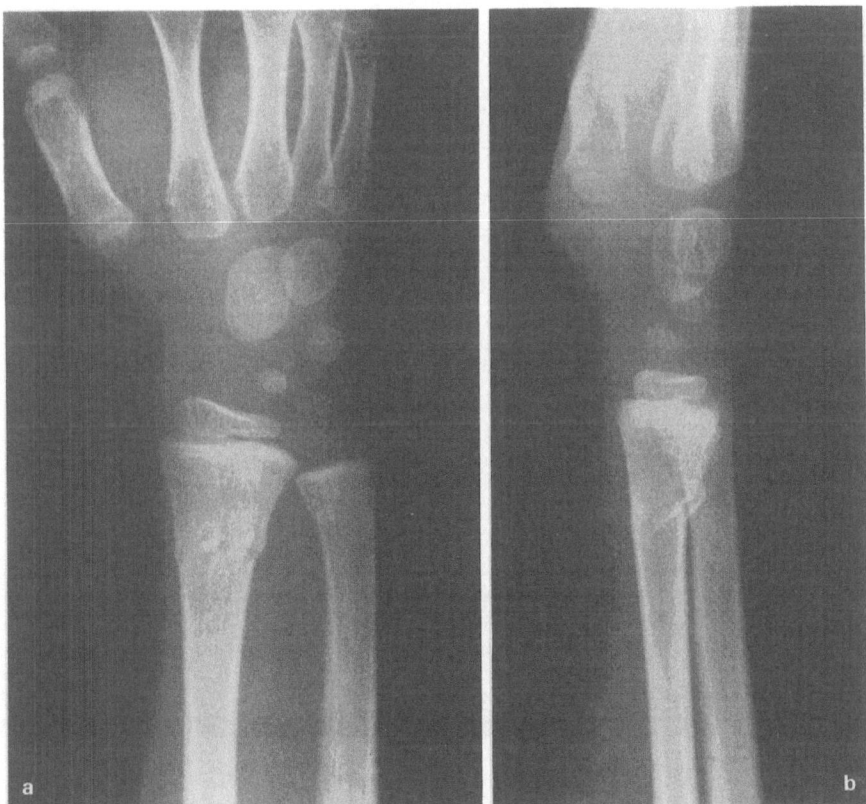

Fig. 3.5.a Greenstick fracture at the lower end of the radius. **b** The crumpled bone is always best seen in the lateral view of this common fracture.

6) *Stress fractures*. Repeated small insults of trauma may cause a break in just part of the bone diameter, along lines of strain. Sports injuries are a good example, e.g. in running, the pounding delivered to the lower limbs can result in such stress fractures (Fig. 3.6).

7) *Pathological fractures*. This is the name given to fractures through bone tumours, most commonly secondary deposits. There are two clues when such a patient presents. (a) *Clinical*—the trauma causing the injury was probably a minimal, everyday activity. (b) *Radiological*—extensive bone destruction is seen all around the fractured part.

8) *Partial fractures in metabolic bone disease*. These lesions bridge topics 6 and 7 above: the breaks are incomplete stress fractures through the abnormal, weakened bone. They are illustrated under *"Osteomalacia"* below, but also occur in Paget's disease.

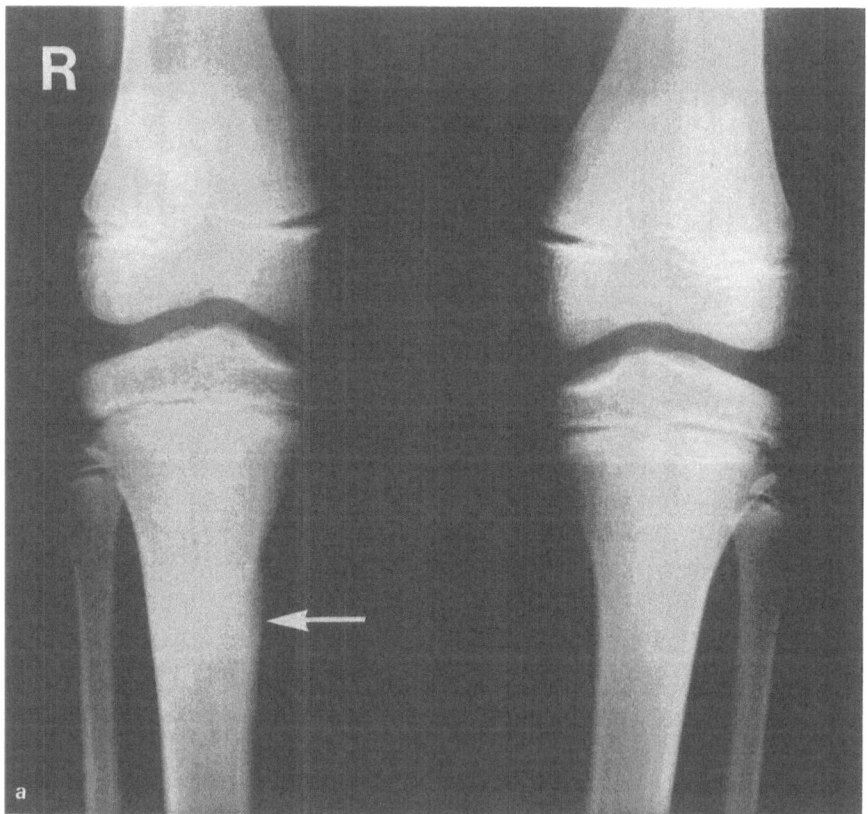

Fig. 3.6.a Stress fracture at the upper end of the right tibia. This film has been taken 2 weeks after the insult, allowing time for new bone ("periosteal reaction") to become visible at the site of injury (*arrow*). **b** A nuclear medicine scan, using a bone-seeking radio-isotope shows the increased activity at the fracture site. There is, of course, also considerable activity at the growing ends of normal bones.

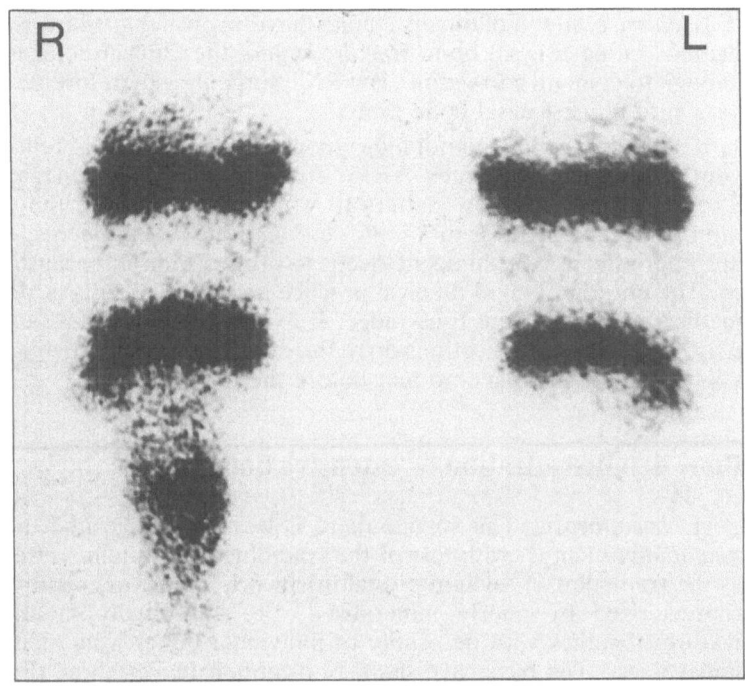

▲ Fig. 3.6.b

Don'ts

1) *Rib fractures.* Cracks in ribs are common but generally of no importance in themselves to further management. The patient with a bruised chest wall may benefit from local measures such as strapping. The single but vital point of x-raying him is to find out whether the underlying lung has been damaged. The request note should therefore read "chest wall trauma: ?pneumothorax or haemothorax". In other words, rib fractures need a chest, not rib, x-ray. This holds good a few days later too, when you may want to check whether your now feverish patient has developed a pneumonia in a poorly ventilated lobe under the hurt rib.

An exception is the badly crushed patient (usually as a result of a traffic injury) who cannot move part of his chest wall at all because a series of ribs are broken in two places along their course. Such a "flail chest" cannot work as a ventilatory device, and you certainly want to know about the extent of the rib injuries as well as the damage to the underlying lung.

2) *Ankle injuries.* Sprains are very common here, and only rarely accompanied by a bony injury. The simple rule in adults is: "no swelling—no fracture". There is no point in x-raying a recently injured but unswollen ankle in an adult.

If you *do* suspect a more severe injury because the ankle is swollen, do not ask for "ankle-and-foot x-rays" like "fish-and-chips", unless there are also clinical signs of an additional foot injury.

3) *Nasal bones*. Follow-up studies have shown that there is no value in demonstrating a nasal bone fracture unless the clinical deformity is severe enough to demand correction. The ENT surgeon is therefore the only proper person to request nasal bone x-rays.

4) *"Medico-legal"*. Do not hide ignorantly under this umbrella like some of your established colleagues. There are very good medico-legal reasons for x-rays: when it properly matters to your patient to have the extent of his injuries documented for the future, e.g. in industrial accidents. Poor reasons are where the doctor thinks he needs to protect himself because the law says so. The criteria of good medical practice are proper habits as defined by the medical profession, not by a judge. If expert medical witnesses can say that reasonable clinical indications drive the need to x-ray a particular patient, the young doctor need have no fear before the law.

Bone demineralization or extensive bone loss

1) *Osteoporosis*. This means there is less total bone than normal, i.e. a *quantitative* change, with loss of the (radiolucent) protein scaffolding as well as the (radiodense) calcium crystal brickwork. The x-ray picture is therefore characterized by poorly mineralized, i.e. abnormally radiolucent, bony texture, together with deformity of individual bones which have given way under stress. The biconcave shape of osteoporotic vertebrae (Fig. 3.7) is the best known deformity. Osteoporosis is a universal ageing phenomenon, but can be set into a galloping pace by various conditions, notably Cushing's syndrome and steroid therapy.

2) *Osteomalacia*. This is a *qualitative* bone change, with inadequate mineralization (calcium crystal deposition) in a normal protein scaffolding. In young children deprived of vitamin D, *rickets* is a synonym. The x-ray picture is therefore also one of abnormally radiolucent bone, but there are additional characteristic features. In children with rickets there are deformities of the growth plate (metaphysis), more easily illustrated than described (Fig. 3.8). Adults show partial fractures (Looser's zones, Milkman's fractures) across part of the diameter of bony parts (Fig. 3.9).

3) *Hyperparathyroidism*. Cortical bone resorption leads to characteristic cortical erosions (Fig. 3.10). Unfortunately most patients with the disease, whether primary or secondary, do *not* show these lesions, though it is always worth looking for them.

4) *Metastases*. Extensive bone deposits can give rise to a picture of widespread demineralization. Myeloma is a good example (Fig. 3.11).

Fig. 3.8. The metaphyses (growth plates) at the lower ends of the radius and ulna are splayed and fuzzy in this child—compare with the normal metaphyses in Fig. 3.3. This is the diagnostic picture of rickets.

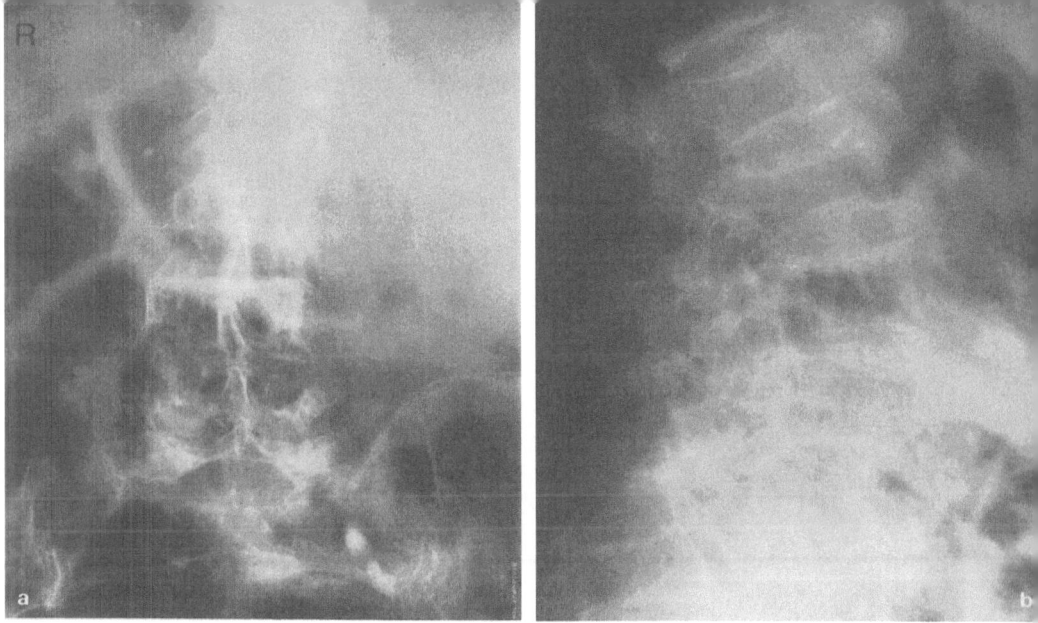

Fig. 3.7.a and **b** Severe osteoporosis in an elderly patient. Vertebral bodies have become compressed into a biconcave shape. Such x-rays always appear to be of poor quality—the reason is loss of bone, with inevitable lack of radiographic contrast (no calcium!).

Fig. 3.8.

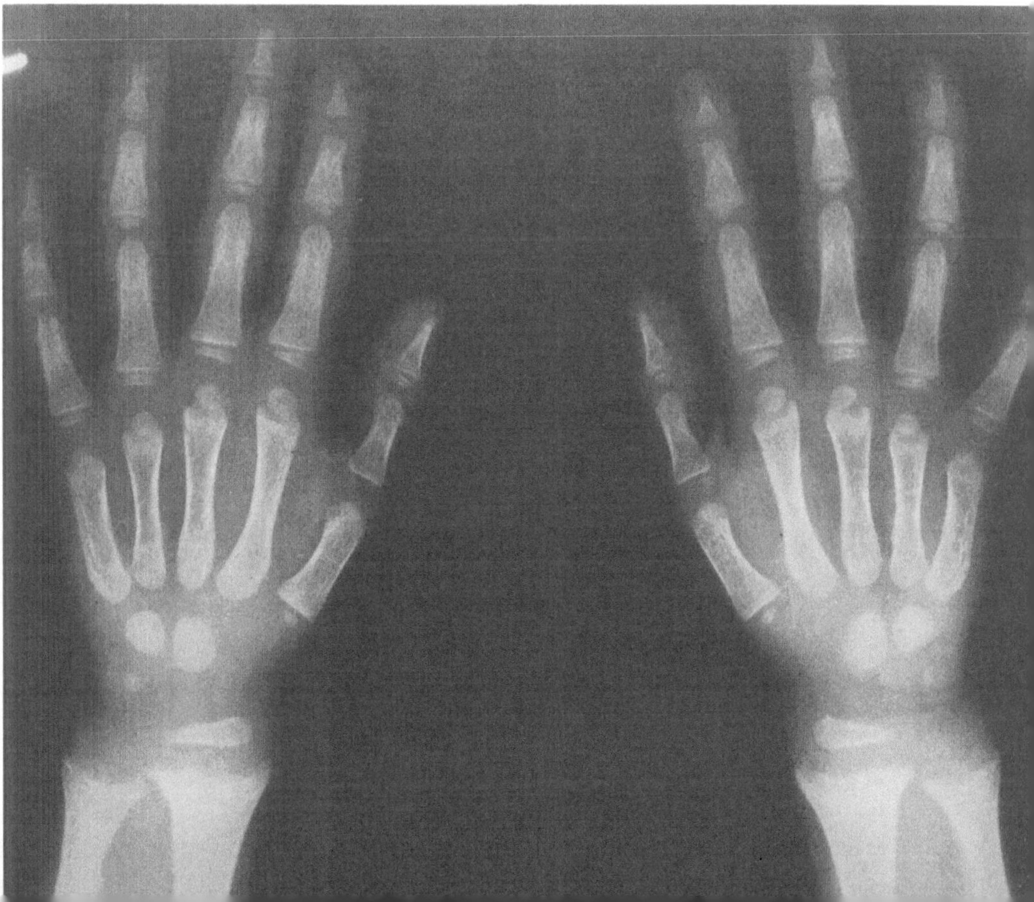

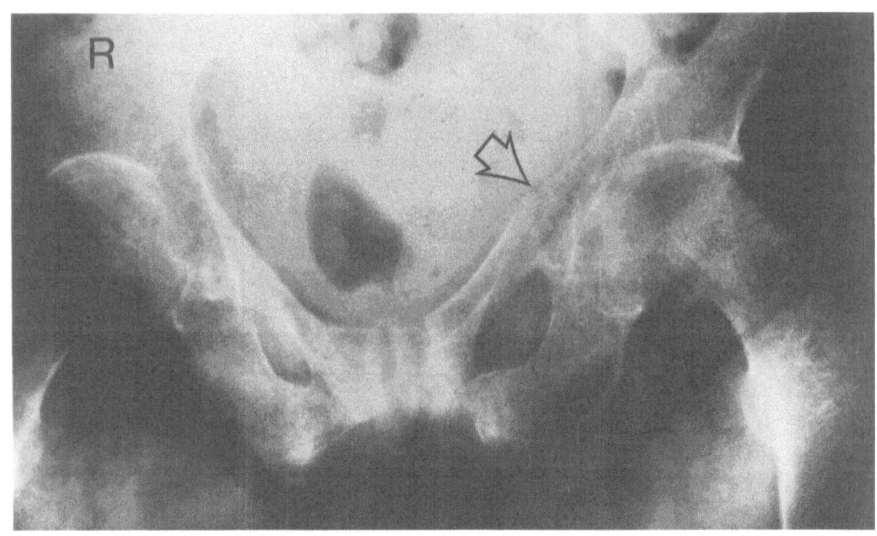

Fig. 3.9. The pelvis in this elderly patient is deformed, and an *arrow* points to the fract opposite the left acetabulum. The radiograph appears poor because the bone has lost so m calcium. This is the diagnostic picture of adult osteomalacia.

Fig. 3.10.a ▼

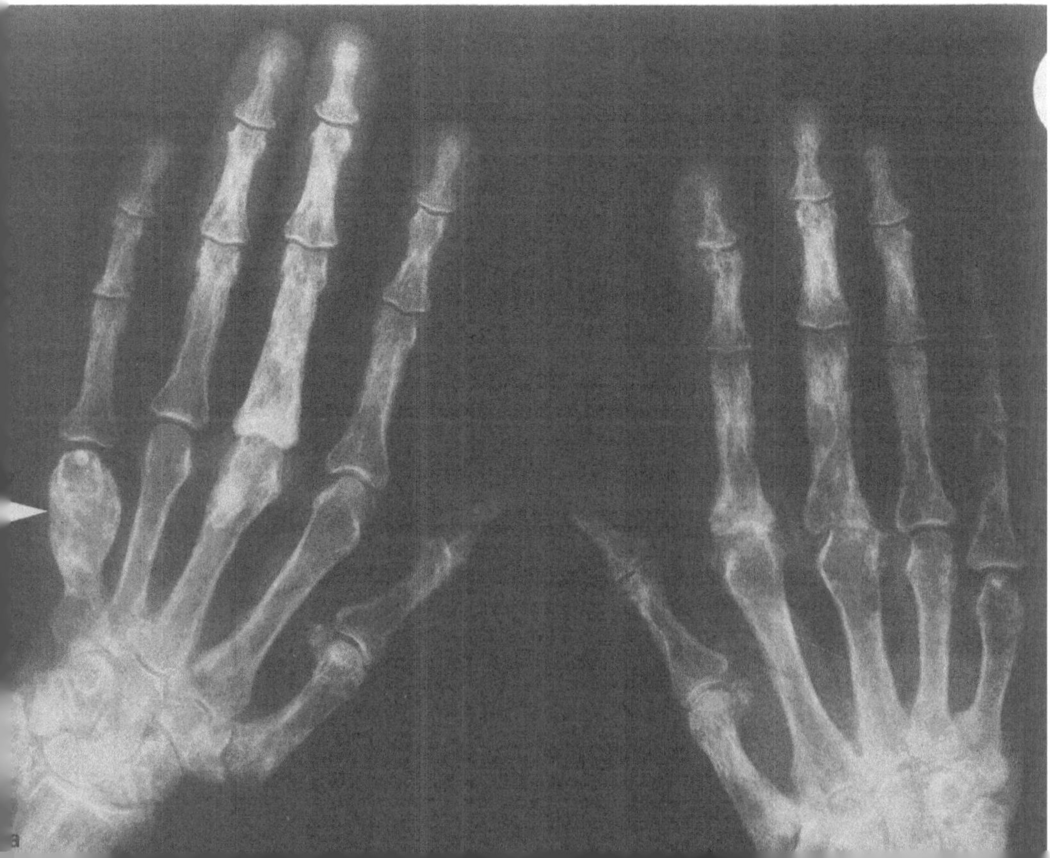

Fig. 3.10.a and **b** Another patient with very marked calcium loss from the skeleton, but here there are quite different associated abnormalities. Note how the dense cortical outline of bone has been lost in **b**—compare with the normal adult picture in Fig. 3.14. There are additional abnormalities deforming the interior of many bones here, most obviously in a 5th metacarpal (*arrow*). Cortical erosions are the hallmark of hyperparathyroidism, and the additional little-finger deformity ("brown tumour") makes this primary hyperparathyroidism.

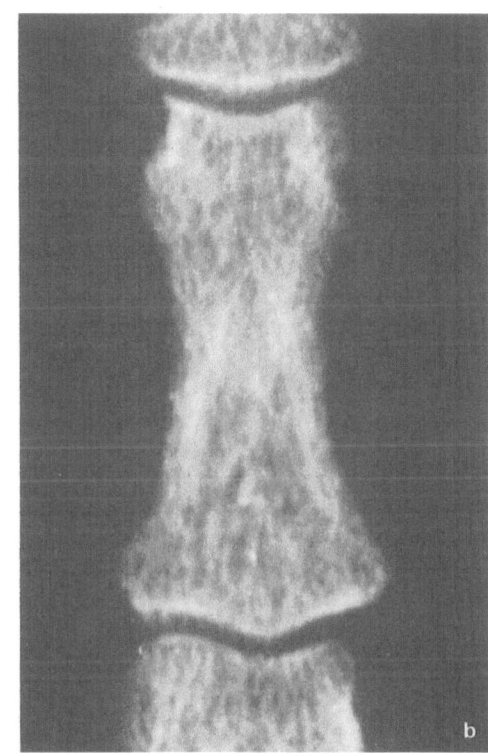
b

Fig. 3.11. There are multiple destructive lesions in the vault of this patient's skull—multiple myeloma. ▼

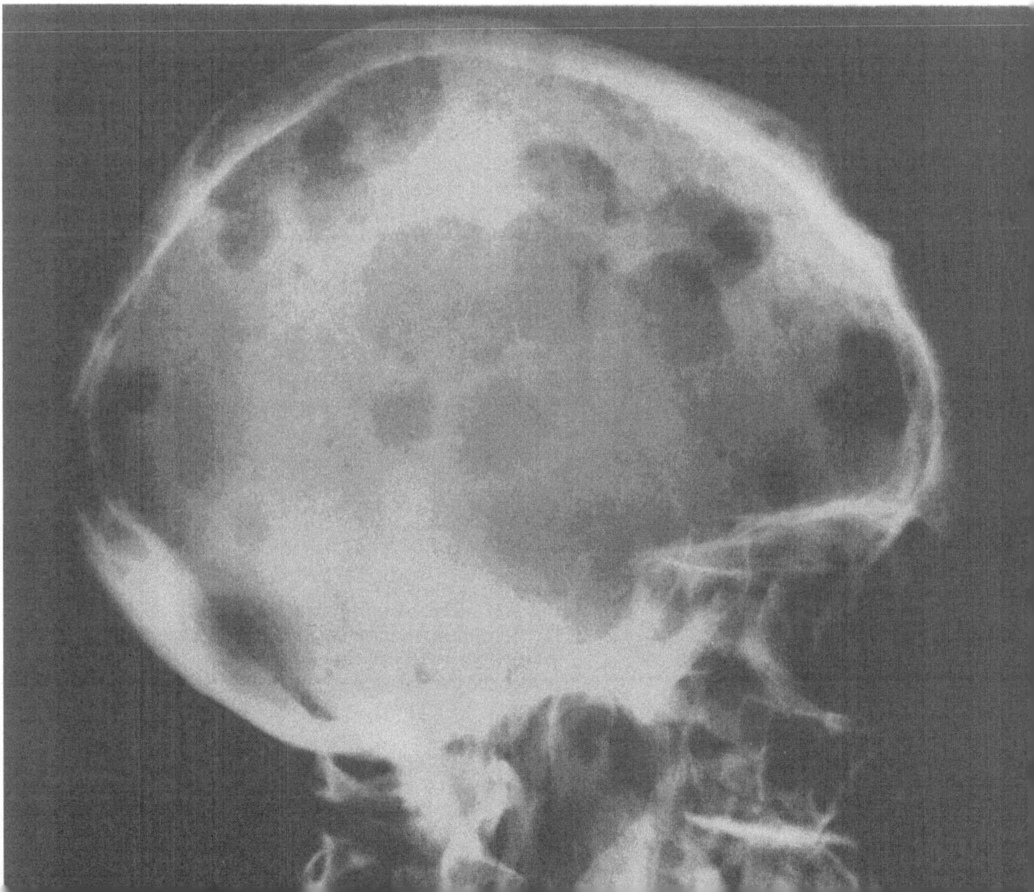

Radionuclide versus x-ray studies

A bone radiograph is a summation picture of the many superimposed calcium crystal bricks which make up an osseous building. It therefore represents *structure*, and is good at answering some questions, but quite hopeless at others. "Is there a crack in the building, with daylight showing through?"—a radiograph will tell you. "Has every second brick in the building been taken out surreptitiously, but so that the weakened structure still stands?"—a radiograph may look normal, even if almost half the bone traversed by the

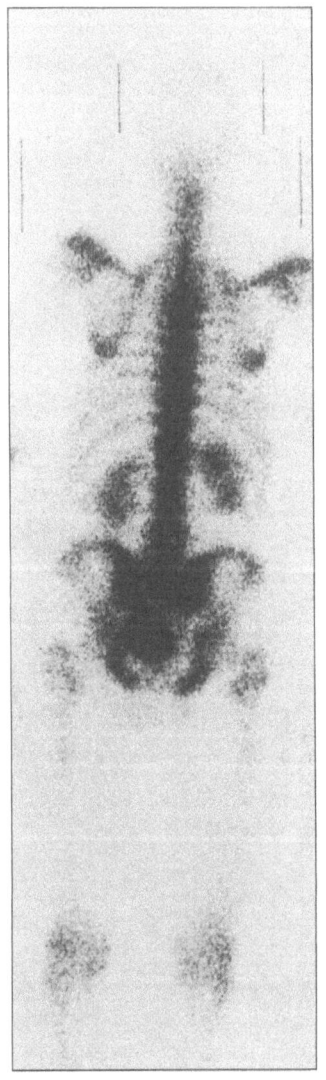

Fig. 3.12. Radio-isotope bone scan, using a technetium-labelled diphosphonate derivative. This is a normal scan—note that the agent is excreted by the kidneys, so lighting up these organs as well as the bladder.

x-ray beam has been removed. Most importantly, the structural study will not reveal the dynamic state of an active tissue like bone. "Is there increased turnover in the building, with all the bricks taken out and replaced much faster than usual?"—you must do a *radionuclide* study of *bone function*.

A radionuclide bone scan hangs a radioactive label, most commonly technetium, onto a molecule involved in bone replacement, now usually a disphosphonate derivative. A gamma-ray picture is obtained some hours later, reflecting normal bone turnover (Fig. 3.12). If metastatic lesions are destroying bone, there will be much greater activity here—"hot spots" (Fig. 3.13).

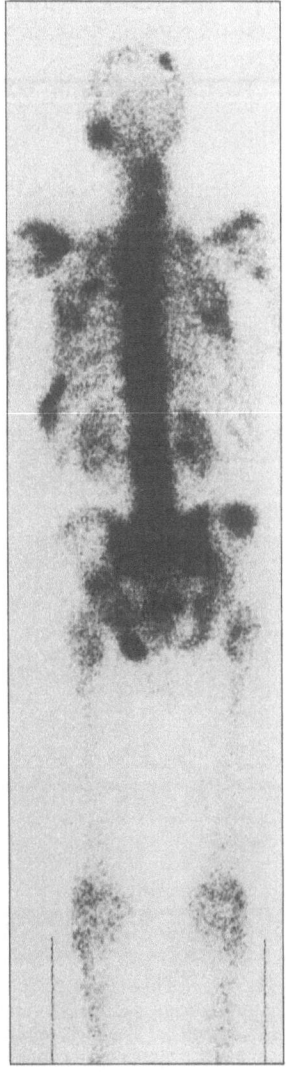

Fig. 3.13. On this bone scan there are multiple "hot spots" throughout the skeleton except in the legs—areas of increased activity denoting increased bone turnover. They mark the multiple bone deposits in this patient with carcinoma of the prostate.

The gamma bone scan is very sensitive—a hot spot will show at once that something is wrong. But it is nonspecific: the lesion may be a deposit, or an infection, or osteoarthritis, or.... Nuclear medicine experts are now quite adept at recognizing some diseases, for instance Paget's. But most of the time, a hot spot discovered during a bone scan will demand at once comparison with a radiograph to check particularly on benign explanations of the finding, e.g. osteoarthritis. If the x-ray picture is normal in a patient suspected of deposits, a malignant lesion is the likely answer, for the radiograph may be weeks or months behind the nuclear medicine study here.

Strategy. If you want to *stage* a patient with a known carcinoma as to deposits, do a gamma bone scan: if it is normal, he/she does not have bony metastases. If you find hot spots, you will need to x-ray the part in question. If a patient presents with *local* symptoms or signs of bone disease, x-ray the part first—a gamma scan may still be needed later, but a radiograph is the obvious first choice.

Parting shot: bone lives! (Fig. 3.14).

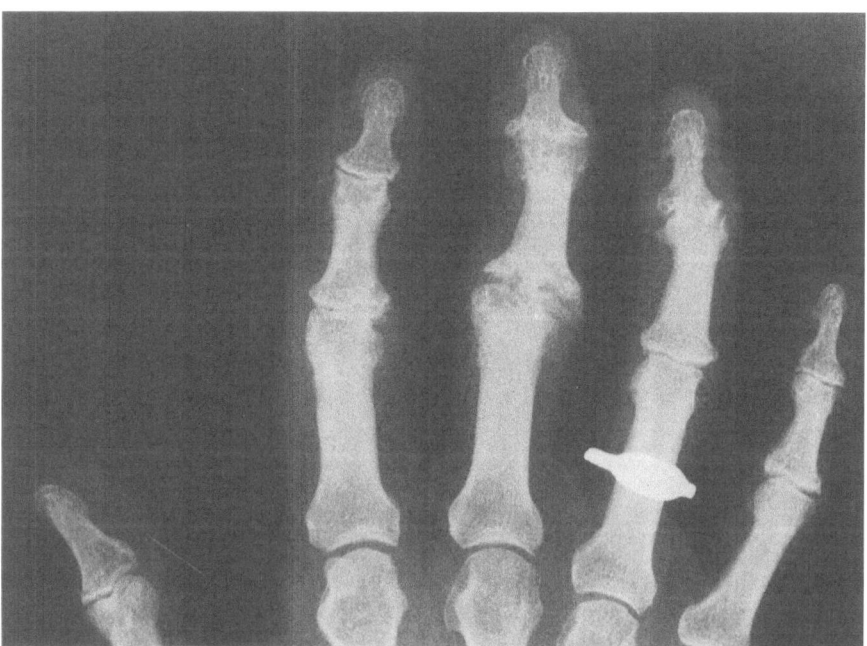

Fig. 3.14. This lady's middle fingers are swollen, and bony excrescences overhang several interphalangeal joints. Several other fingers are also affected. These are Heberden's nodes, or osteoarthritis. The picture reflects a lifetime of remodelling of bone in response to hard use and so-called degenerative changes.

4. The Chest

A lung lesion is usually well demonstrated on chest x-rays on account of the large density difference between a disease process and air in the surrounding normal lung. Although a near-normal chest film can occur in severe chronic bronchitis or pulmonary embolism, a technically satisfactory normal chest x-ray usually excludes lung disease. A clinician who suspects that a patient has pulmonary tuberculosis or bronchial carcinoma will divert his attention elsewhere if the chest x-ray is considered normal. This clinical usefulness has resulted in the chest film being the most commonly requested imaging test.

Technique

The ordinary PA (postero-anterior) chest x-ray (CXR) is a quick and relatively cheap investigation (Fig. 4.1a). Rather than learning cold data about how such a CXR is obtained, it is easier to watch a skilled radiographer in action. Suffice it to say that the suspended inspiration should be maximal, i.e. right dome lower than the inferior aspect of the anterior portion of the right 5th rib. The patient must not be rotated, i.e. vertebral spinous process central between medial ends of clavicles. The film should be correctly exposed and processed, i.e. the lungs must not appear too black (over-exposed) or too pale (underexposed). You should just be able to identify disk spaces of the upper vertebral column on a correctly exposed film—the heart should obscure the disk spaces inferiorly.

Watch out for AP or supine films (the patient may be too ill to come to the department for conventional views)—such films should be clearly labelled. The heart and mediastinum (anterior structures) may appear alarmingly large due to the inevitable magnification. When supine, free pleural fluid will form a thin layer posteriorly and be hard to detect; the diaphragm can be deceptively well defined.

The lateral CXR (Fig. 4.1b) offers a second look at an abnormality suspected on the PA CXR. The lateral CXR will localize the abnormality and confirm that it is truly intrathoracic (avoiding the catastrophe of calling a skin

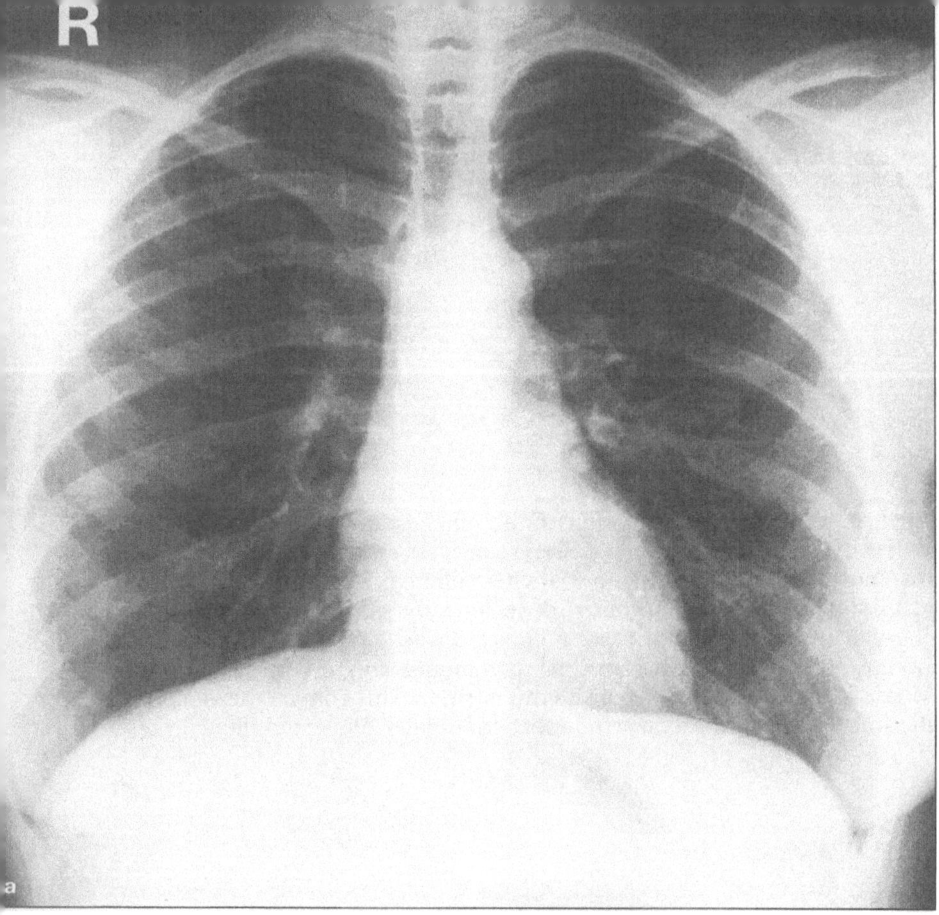

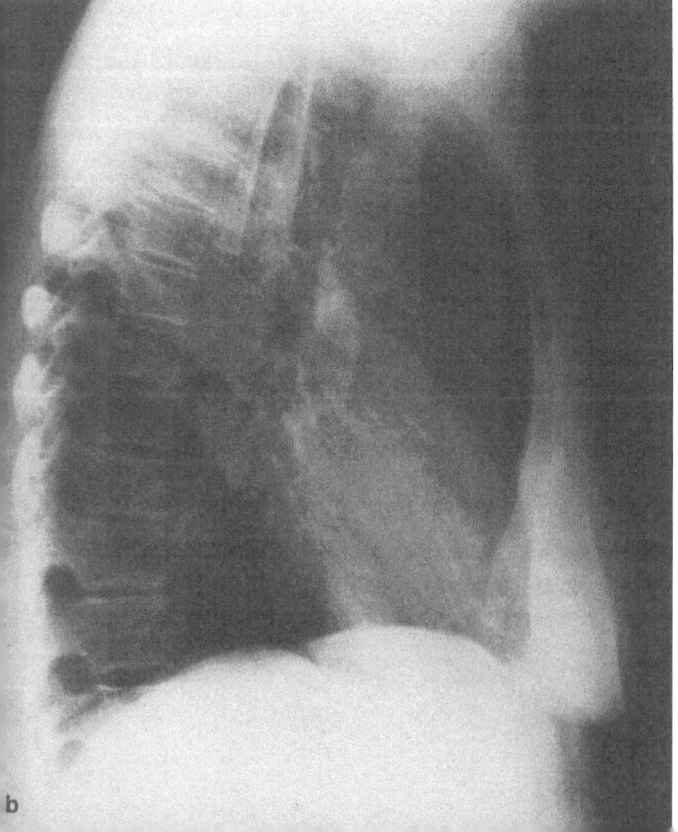

Fig. 4.1.a Normal postero-anterior (PA) chest x-ray.

Fig. 4.1.b Normal lateral chest film. Note how the retrosternal density marries with the retrocardiac density.

lesion an intrathoracic tumour). Radiographers are instructed to perform a lateral CXR when an untoward finding is discovered on the PA view, and to obtain advice in doubtful cases. Accordingly, a lateral CXR should probably not be requested as a routine. It will, however, be needed to identify cardiac valvular calcification. It is a great help when assessing the hila (the vascular root shadows) and allows identification of the oblique fissures. Occasionally it will reveal an abnormality when the PA CXR is entirely normal. Such a lesion will usually be in one of the hidden areas of the PA CXR: the anterior mediastinum, behind the heart, in the posterior costophrenic recess (below the dome on the PA view). As a rough-and-ready rule, ask for a lateral CXR in addition to the PA film when:

1) There are abnormal physical signs in the chest
2) You suspect a mediastinal/hilar abnormality (sarcoidosis/lymphoma)
3) Valvular calcification is a possibility.

The penetrated PA CXR is really a misnomer; strictly speaking it is an overexposed PA CXR. It is often needed for cardiac patients as valvular calcification and pacing wires may be seen. Signs of left atrial enlargement may be more evident on an overexposed film: the main bronchi may be splayed at the carina, or the posterior enlargement of the left atrium may be seen as an additional shadow just within the right heart border. Splaying of the carina and distortion of the trachea may also be caused by tumours, and thus an overexposed film may be of value if lymphoma or carcinoma of the bronchus is suspected — especially if there is any possibility of stridor.

Occasionally specialized views are needed. A film exposed in expiration will accentuate the trapped pleural air in a pneumothorax (see Fig. 2.1). This diagnosis can be made on the standard PA film by the hairline lung edge, with increased blackening and an absence of lung markings lateral to this hairline. The expiration film may demonstrate mediastinal shift in a patient with unilateral air trapping, due to ball valve accumulation in a partially obstructed lung or lobe (tumour or foreign body, commonly a peanut). Mediastinal swing is usually easier to determine at fluoroscopy (watching the x-ray image on a television monitor). Fluoroscopy is a quick method of confirming the presence or absence of an opacity suspected on the PA view. Fluoroscopy can also help in assessing a high hemidiaphragm: does the dome move normally (i.e. congenital weakness), does it move paradoxically (i.e. the wrong way: phrenic nerve lesion) or is it immobile (subphrenic abscess)? Sometimes a lordotic (apical) view is useful to gain more information about the apex of the lung—a prime site for tuberculosis and one which can be obscured by the clavicle on a standard PA CXR.

Tomograms

By moving the source of x-rays and the film during the exposure in a related manner, with the patient as fulcrum, it is possible to focus down on a particular plane of the body, blurring out overlying structures. The body-

35

section radiograph thus obtained is known as a tomogram. This technique is very helpful in assessing hilar structures (hilar tomograms) and possible small pulmonary metastases (whole-lung tomograms). Tomograms are particularly helpful in deciding whether or not an abnormality is present when there is still some doubt after routine views. Thus, when on the PA and lateral CXR a hilar shadow is considered "prominent", the radiologist may request hilar tomograms to establish whether there is additional nodal material present, or whether the normal vascular structures are unusually large. On the whole, the fashion of using tomography to gain further information about a definite abnormality is declining, although signs such as cavitation may be demonstrated. Since histology is required for the diagnosis, either fibre-optic bronchoscopy or needle biopsy under screening control is now advocated if sputum examinations fail to reveal the responsible organism or tumour.

Computed tomography

Computed tomography is a new technique and its role in the investigation of intrathoracic disease is still being evaluated. A computer-reconstructed cross-sectional image is obtained from the data available after numerous narrow fan-beam x-ray exposures have passed through the body to specialized detectors. The number of exposures is related to the number of detectors used, which in turn is related to the number of pixels in the image matrix (usually 256×256). This image can be displayed on a television monitor in several ways, depending on what sort of tissue is under scrutiny. The total range of tissue attenuation is arbitrarily spread from air (-1000 units) through water (0) to bone at $+1000$ and above. The unit is named the Hounsfield after the inventor of EMI CT scanning. A wide range at a negative level (-800) is used to view the lung parenchyma (Fig. 4.2a), while a soft tissue density level (about $+40$) is required to view the structures of the mediastinum (Fig. 4.2b). Computed tomography is now widely considered to be the optimal method of investigating patients with mediastinal abnormalities. It may prove helpful in assessing operability of thoracic tumours. A characteristic peripheral soft tissue density lesion seen at CT is much the earliest manifestation of a pulmonary secondary deposit (Fig. 4.3). Deposits must be differentiated from granulomatous lesions—less of a problem in the United Kingdom than in the United States where histoplasmosis is widespread. At the end of evaluation it is likely that body CT will find its major role for disease within the abdomen and mediastinum. In the chest a 5-cm diameter lesion should be clearly seen by a conventional PA CXR due to nature's own contrast medium—air. In the abdomen more sophisticated techniques will frequently be required to demonstrate such a lesion.

Interpretation

Students frequently ask us to instruct them how to "go through" the interpretation of a chest film. In practice the radiologist makes horrendous short cuts. When referred a patient with "?pneumonia", the lungs are

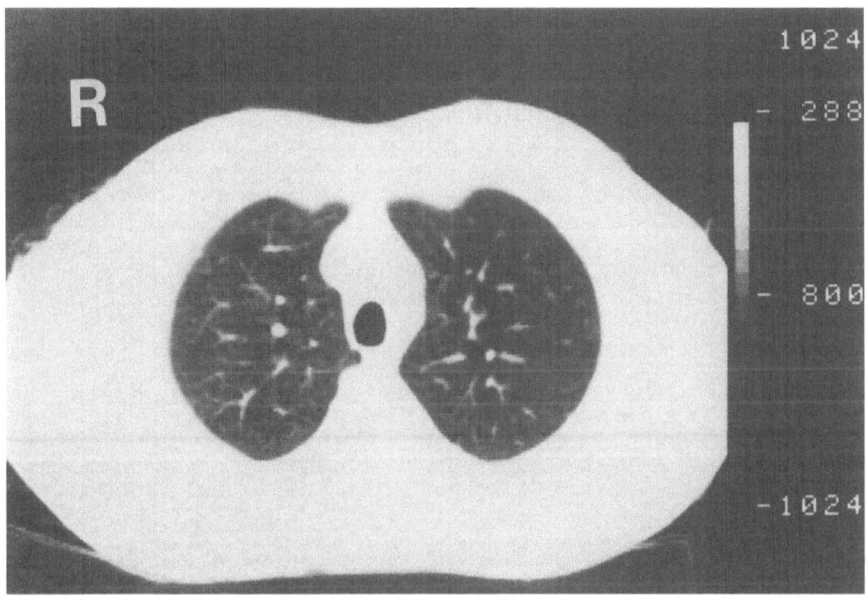

Fig. 4.2.a CT scan through upper chest. Normal lung vessels shown at a negative level (−800).

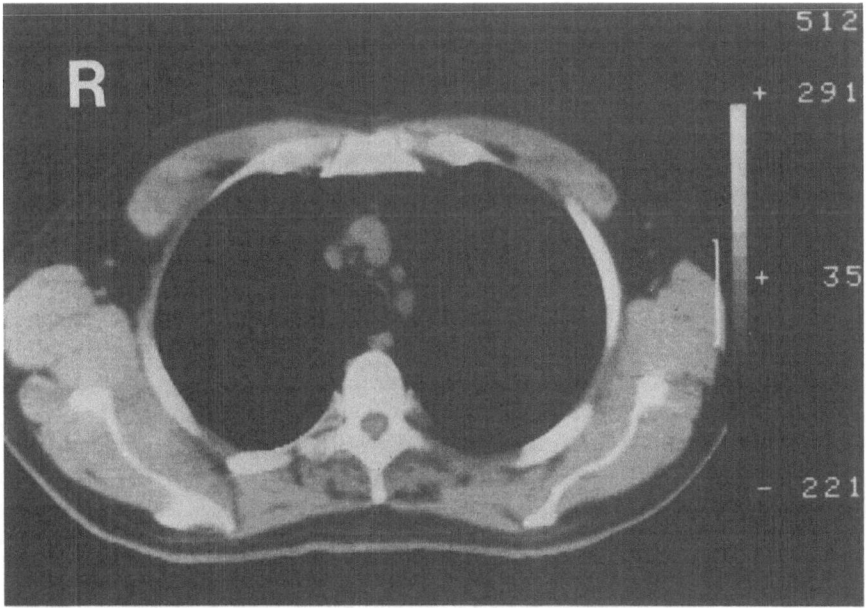

Fig. 4.2.b The same scan viewed at a soft tissue level (+35). The great vessels are clearly seen within the superior mediastinum.

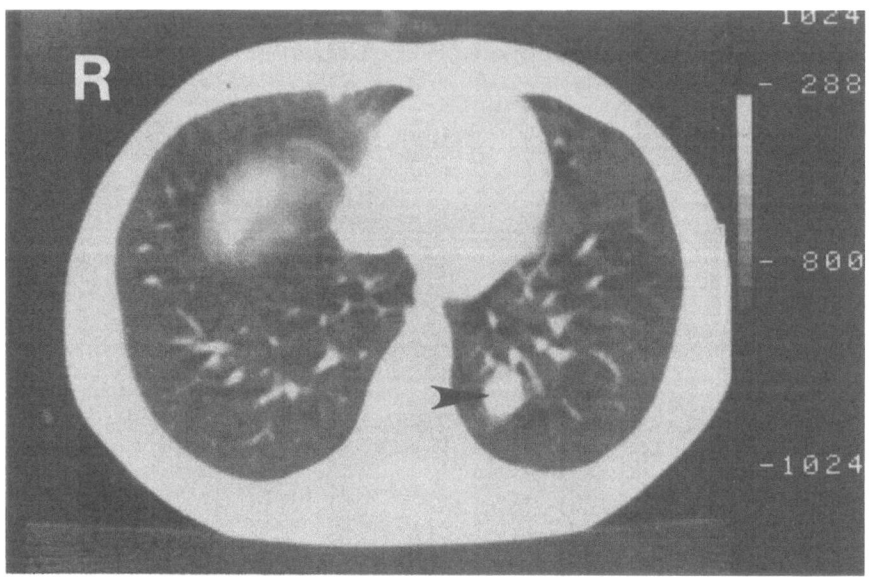

Fig. 4.3. Secondary deposit (*arrow*) in a patient with a primary teratoma of the testis. This was hidden behind the heart on the PA CXR. The opacity in the right lung is the top of the right dome.

carefully inspected, but only a cursory glance will be given to the clavicle. The reverse would apply to a patient on renal dialysis where detailed examination of the outer rims of the clavicles might reveal changes of hyperparathyroidism or renal osteodystrophy. But when starting to interpret chest films, some orderly scheme is required; each radiologist will advise and each physician will adopt his own personal scheme. The necessary facts may be obtained from standard texts (Simon 1971; Fraser and Paré 1977). A thumbnail scheme might run as follows.

1) Technical factors—patient's name, right/left labelling, rotation, degree of inspiration and exposure.
2) Heart/mediastinum—size, shape, position, clarity of outline, calcification, trachea + main bronchi, additional retrocardiac shadow? (Fig. 4.4).
3) Hilar (lung root) shadows—level, size, density.
4) Lungs—general opaqueness (whiteness)/lucency (blackness), normal vascular shadows, ?additional shadows (nodules/lines/confluent), difficult areas (paraspinal/apices/peripheral/below dome in posterior costophrenic sulcus).
5) Domes of diaphragm—level, clarity, sharpness of costophrenic angles, gastric air bubble, ?free air under dome.
6) Skeletal—ribs/scapulae/clavicles/vertebrae.
7) Soft tissues—breast, nipple, muscles, skin lesions, artefacts from clothes/hair.

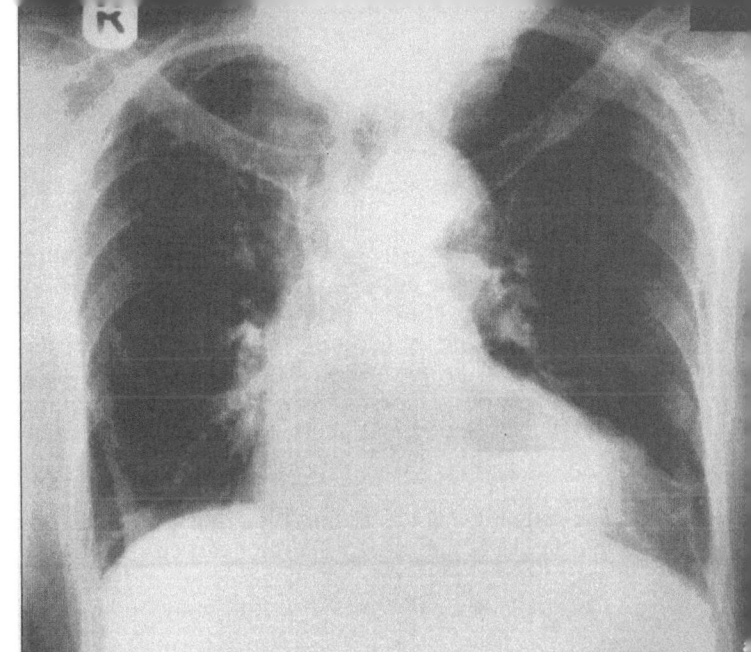

Fig. 4.4.a Fluid level within the cardiac shadow indicates likely hiatus hernia (incarcerated stomach behind the heart). **b** Diagnosis confirmed by lateral view. Air/fluid level well seen behind the heart. Note severe kyphosis in this elderly patient.

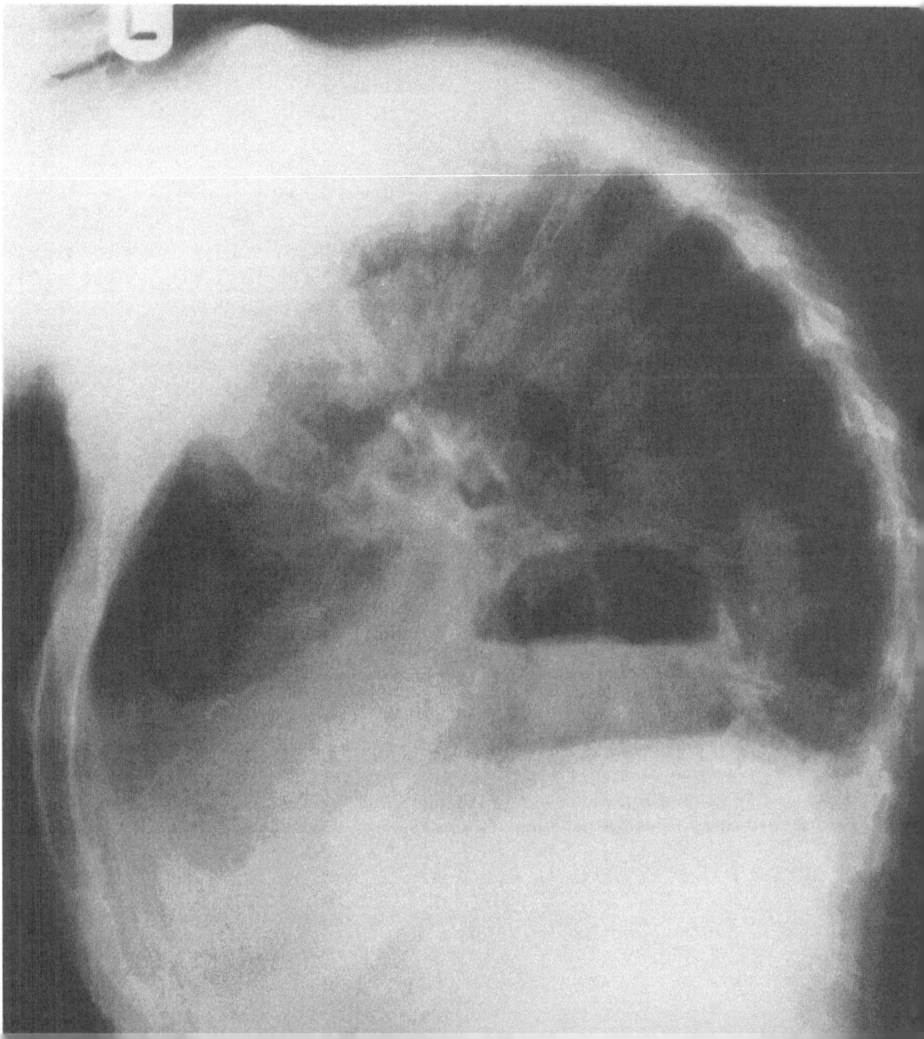

Problems

Big heart

The adult heart is enlarged if, on a standard PA film, its transverse span is 15.5 cm. It may be enlarged (on radiological grounds) at less than 15.5 cm *if* there is evidence (from a previous radiograph) that it has increased by 1.5 cm or more. The widely quoted cardiothoracic ratio is less helpful, because the thorax shrinks in old age so that a normal-sized heart may occupy 50% or more of the thorax. Assessment of heart size in infants is also difficult as the normal heart (aided and abetted by the thymus) may seem alarmingly large (Fig. 4.5); such films will often be taken supine and magnification may play a part.

The radiologically large heart is a dilated heart. Hypertrophy of a ventricle alone should not affect the overall heart size, and even assessment of specific chamber dilatation on radiological grounds is fraught with difficulties. Occasionally the enlarged left atrium may be identified (Fig. 4.6). Eccentric

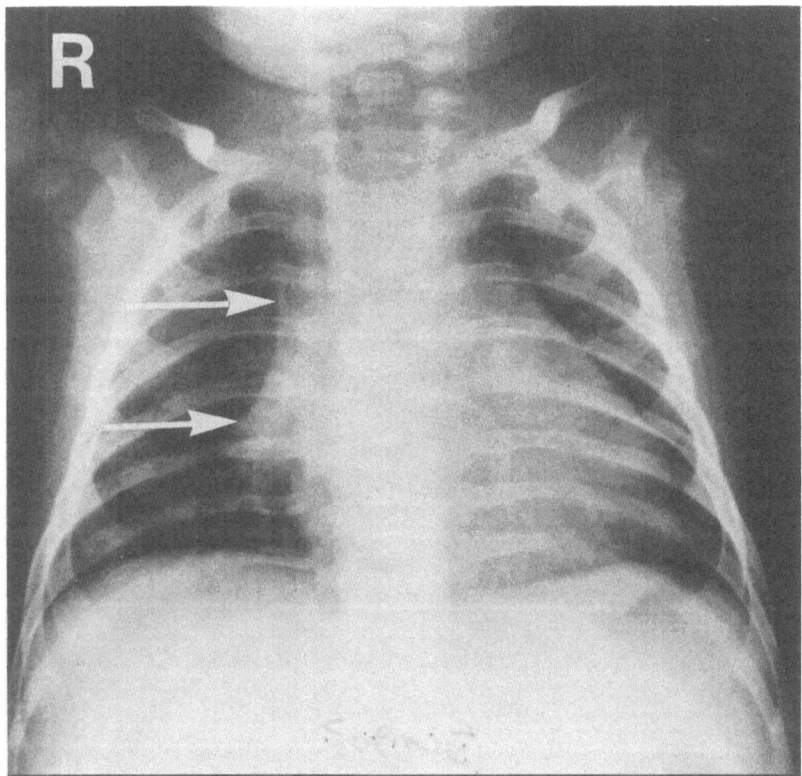

Fig. 4.5. Normal heart in an infant (supine film). Note the sharp outline of the thymus on the right (*arrows*). This has been likened to a sail.

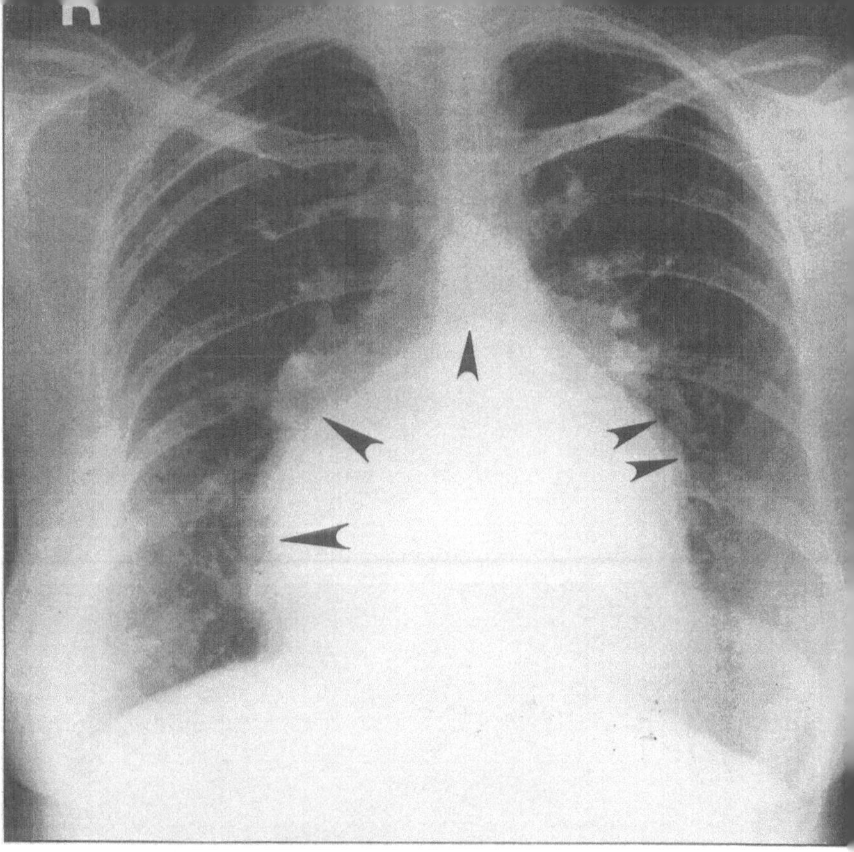

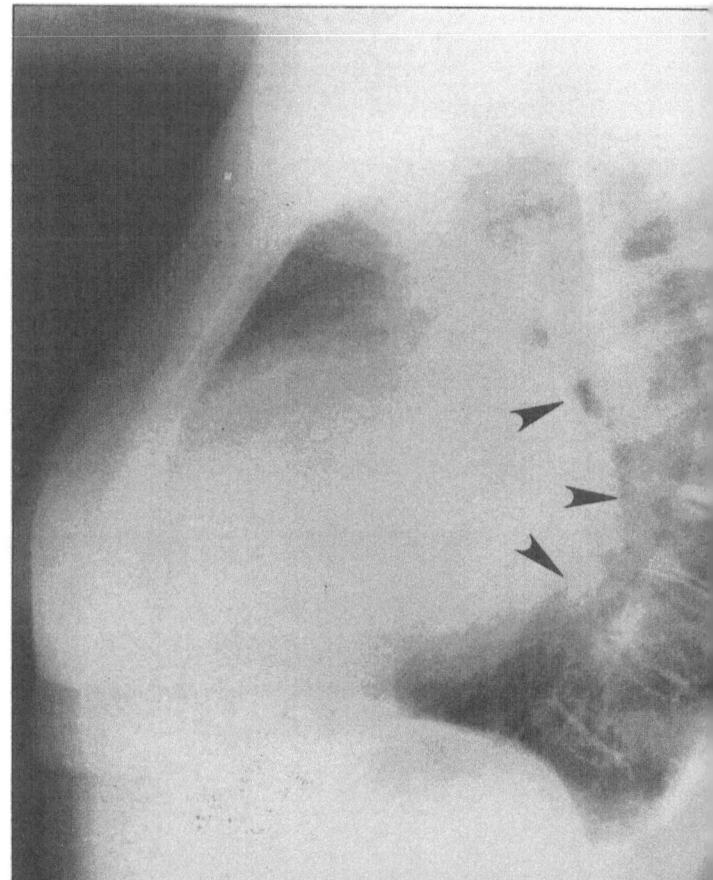

Fig. 4.6.a Mitral valve disease; PA view. The large left atrium is outlined (*arrows*). Note the splaying of the carina. Left atrial appendage enlargement (*double arrows*) is a particularly helpful feature. **b** Lateral film reveals the *posterior* left atrial enlargement (*arrows*).

cardiac enlargement can provide a clue of a ventricular aneurysm (Fig. 4.7), but a similar "boot-shaped" configuration can arise from the altered haemodynamics in some congenital cardiac conditions. Usually more than one chamber is dilated when the heart is radiologically enlarged. Sometimes when the cardiac shadow is considerably enlarged (17+ cm) it may appear nearly spherical. Possibilities include generalized cardiomyopathy or a pericardial effusion. Ultrasound should readily differentiate, allowing quick recognition of the free pericardial fluid.

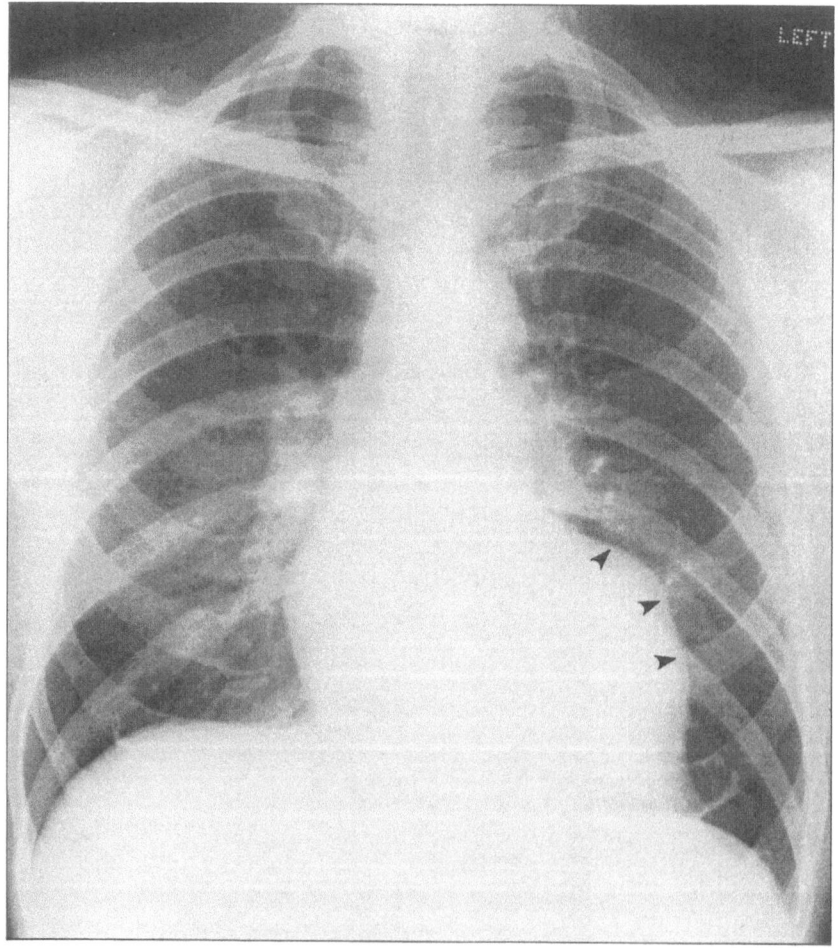

Fig. 4.7. Localized left ventricular enlargement (*arrows*) characteristic of aneurysm.

Wide mediastinum

Sadly, there are no figures to allow measurement here, and assessment has to be subjective. Do not be confused by misleading appearances on rotated or poor inspiratory films. With increasing age the aorta elongates and becomes ectatic (generally dilated). This leads to aortic tortuosity which may be accentuated by increasing kyphosis. Thus the aorta alone can be responsible for an alarmingly wide mediastinum. The innominate artery can also become ectatic and produce a familiar right superior mediastinum shadow (Fig. 4.8). Against this background the recognition of a dissecting thoracic aortic aneurysm may be difficult. If any patient has chest pain, think of it; if a patient has chest pain and a wide mediastinum (even on an AP film), look hard for evidence of left pleural fluid (blood from leakage) or unequal pulses.

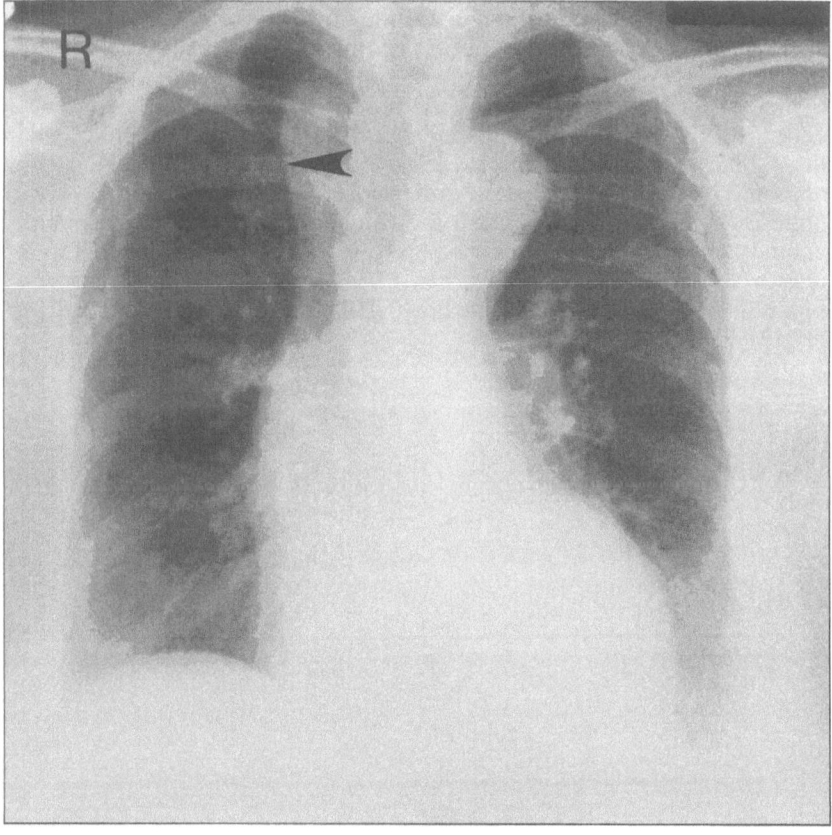

Fig. 4.8. Right superior mediastinal shadow (*arrow*) caused by a wide tortuous innominate artery in an elderly patient. There is generalized aortic dilatation and unfolding causing a wide mediastinum and a prominent aortic knuckle. All these features are accentuated because of slight rotation (left shoulder forward).

The usual worries in a patient with a suspiciously wide mediastinum rest between nodal enlargement and anterior mediastinal tumours. The nodal enlargement may be secondary to a peripheral lung neoplasm (maybe tiny), or part of a more generalized process such as tuberculosis, sarcoid or lymphoma. The anterior mediastinal tumour (*t*hymoma, *t*eratoma, *t*hyroid lesion extending retrosternally) may be best seen on the lateral view: the normal retrosternal lucent region (caused by the lungs meeting anteriorly) is filled by the tumour of soft tissue density—opaque (Fig. 4.9).

Worrying hilar shadows

Questionably abnormal hilar shadows are one of the commonest topics for discussion between clinician and radiologist (and between radiologists). There is the constant anxiety that the questionably prominent hilum may be harbouring the first signs of disease (tumour or tuberculosis for example). A hilum surrounded by additional nodal material (Fig. 4.10) should be more opaque than its counterpart on the normal side. With luck, the diseased hilum will also appear larger, although this may be hard to appreciate. Confusion arises mainly because the size of the arterial and venous structures is variable. The arterial system will enlarge in pulmonary hypertension (remember chronic bronchitis/emphysema is common), when the basal arteries will be enlarged (Fig. 4.11). Although such arterial enlargement should be bilateral, the right basal artery is often easier to see than the left (which may be obscured by the heart border). Furthermore, the left pulmonary artery can be quite prominent even in normal individuals as it hooks up, over and then behind the left main bronchus. So the scene is set for uncertainty in interpretation. The lateral view can be very helpful as nodes may be seen separate from the vascular structures. Hilar tomograms may be needed to resolve such problems.

Fig. 4.9.a Grossly abnormal mediastinal shadow. **b** Lateral view shows filling in of the normal retrosternal lucency. This proves that the bulk of the tumour is in the anterior mediastinum. It proved to be a teratoma.

Fig. 4.9.a ▶

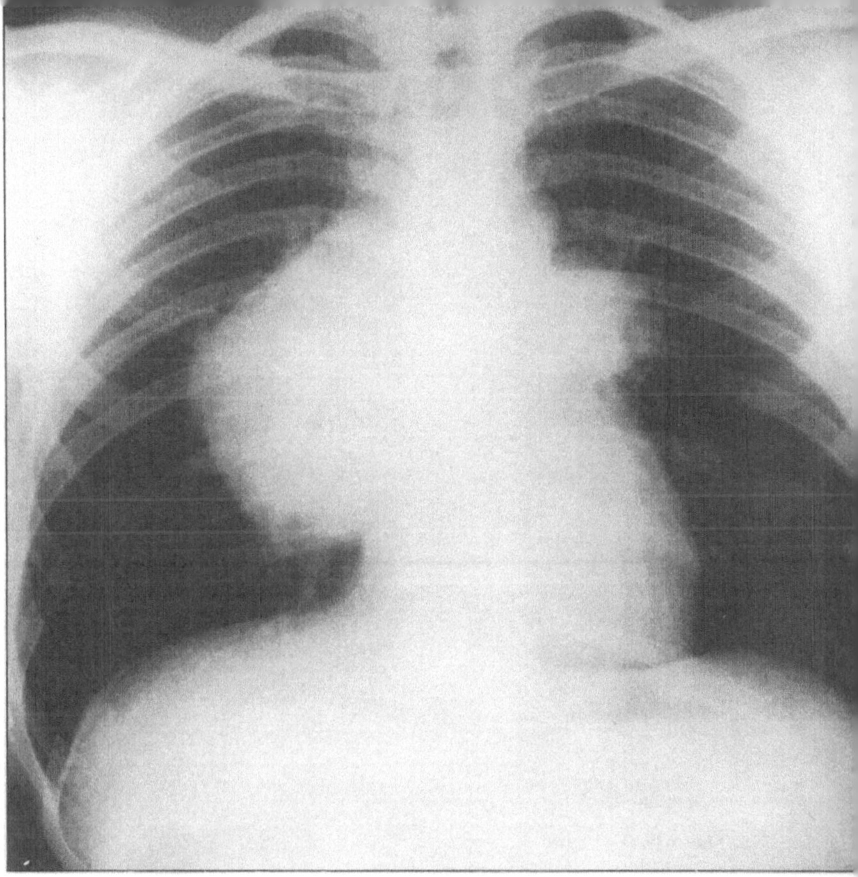

Fig. 4.9.b ▶

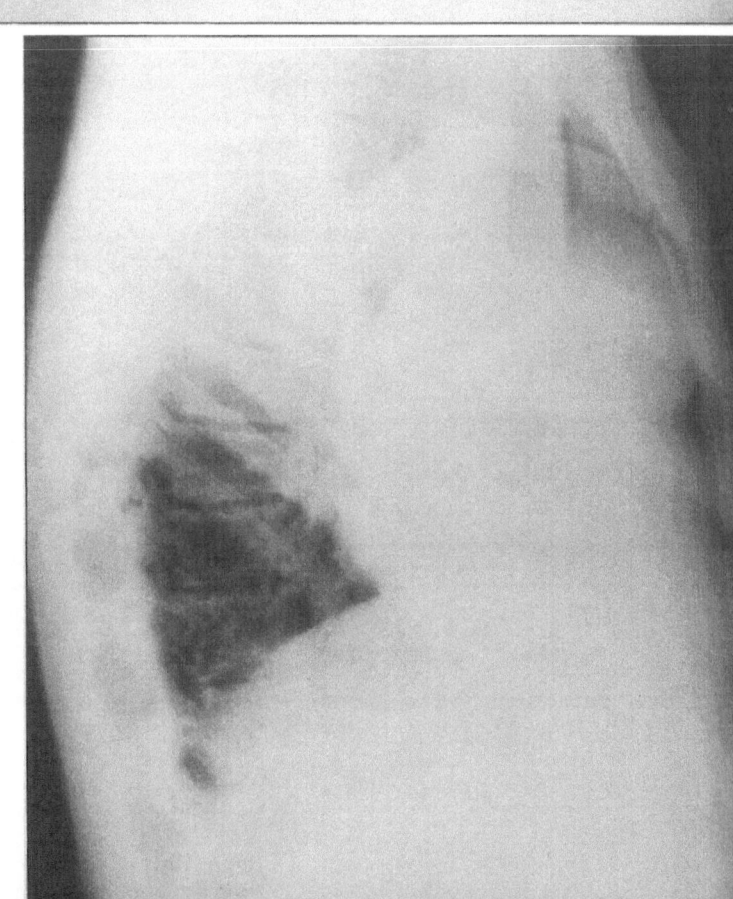

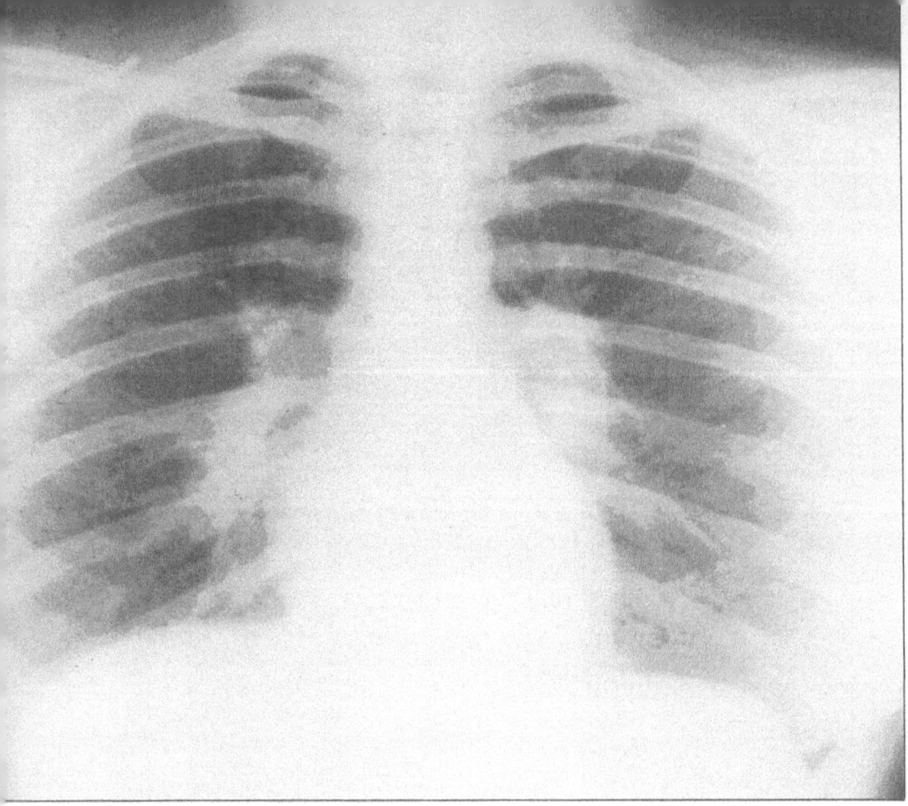

Fig. 4.10 ▲

Fig. 4.11 ▼

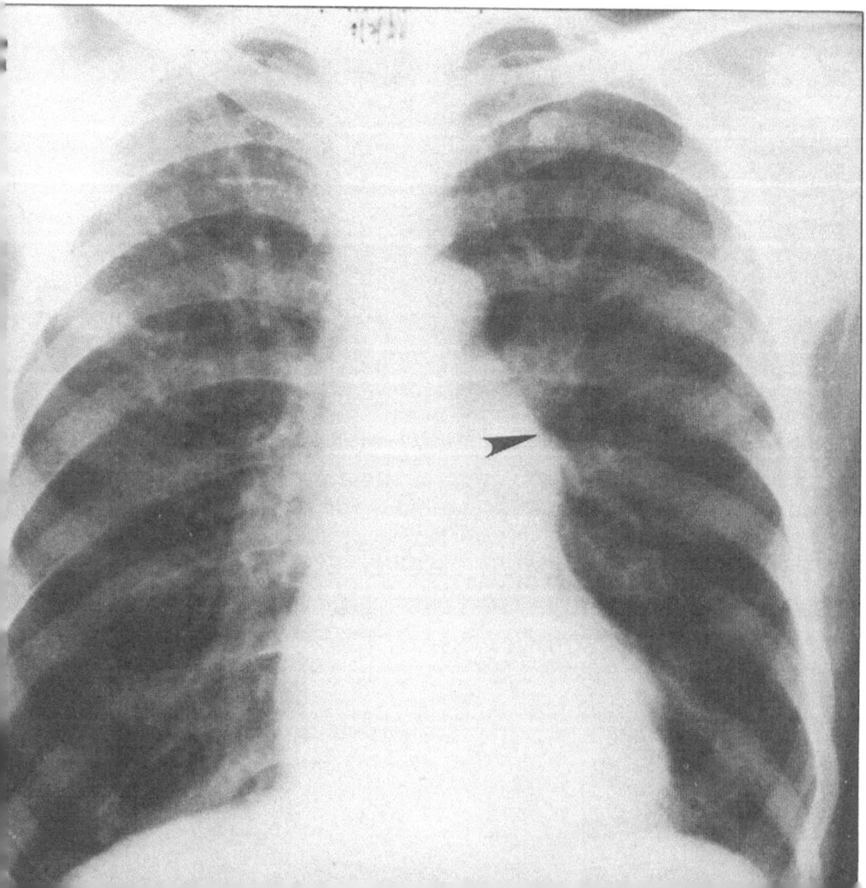

Fig. 4.10. Hilar enlargement in a fit patient presenting with erythema nodosum. Sarcoidosis diagnosed on the basis of this chest x-ray. The hilar enlargement (caused by sarcoid involvement of lymph nodes) is most marked on the left. The right hilum is also abnormal, especially inferiorly.

Lungs

Chest x-rays are often required to establish the presence or absence of consolidation. Any process where the alveoli are filled with fluid can be called consolidation. Such fluid is commonly pus (pneumonia) or transudate (pulmonary oedema); blood or neoplastic cells in the alveoli can sometimes be responsible for consolidation. Confluent fluid-filled alveoli will show up as an opacity while the bronchi, which tend to remain air filled in consolidation, will appear as lucencies within the opaque area. This sign of air-filled bronchi rendered lucent by the fluid-filled alveoli is known as the *air bronchogram* (Fig. 4.12); its recognition allows confident diagnosis of consolidation—but not of its cause. Consolidation due to infection is commonly segmental and

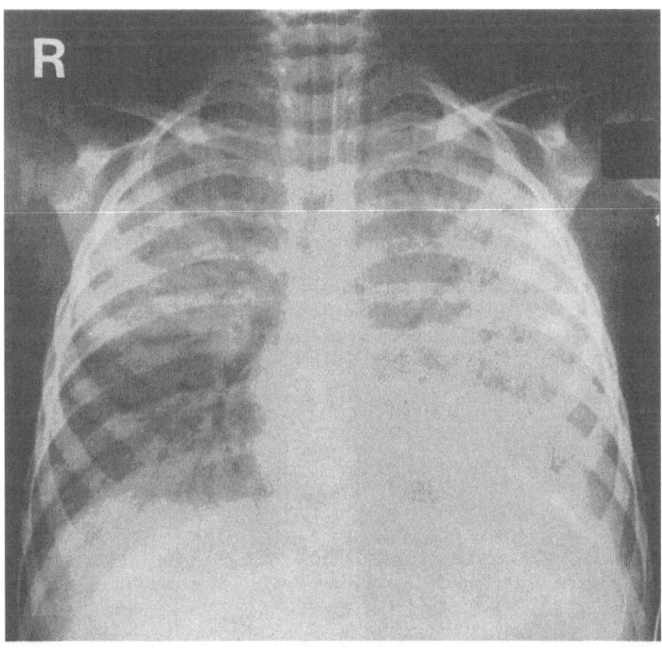

Fig. 4.12. Air bronchogram. This child had overwhelming infection in both lungs and died shortly after this radiograph. The alveoli are full of pus and both lungs are rendered opaque. The bronchial tree (which is still air filled) is clearly seen.

Fig. 4.11. Prominent hilar shadows due to large pulmonary arteries. The pulmonary outflow tract (trunk) is also large (*arrow*). Pulmonary arterial hypertension due to chronic lung disease. Increased perfusion to the upper lobes (less damaged by cigarettes).

the appearances will become familiar. Middle lobe and lingular consolidation may be easily recognized by the lack of definition of the heart border—the normal sharp air/soft tissue (lung/heart) interface will be interrupted (Fig. 4.13). Consolidation abutting fissures or domes will also result in recognizable patterns (Fig. 4.14).

Some practical points on timing. Firstly, it is possible for a CXR to be normal if taken in the first few hours of a pneumonic process. At the other end of the process, the CXR may remain abnormal for a week or more even after clinical improvement following suitable treatment. The resolution of the x-ray signs in elderly patients with pneumonia can be very slow (in the order of months). It is essential to prove that such patients' CXRs return to normal. Occasionally pneumonia may be caused by a predisposing abnormality such as bronchiectasis, aspiration, or bronchial foreign body/tumour. In such instances the pneumonia may not respond to treatment, or may recur in a similar site. But resist the temptation to obtain frequent check CXRs to monitor progress—they will often cause unwarranted alarm to a patient whose clinical progress is satisfactory! About three radiographs should suffice in most patients with straightforward pneumonia: one for diagnosis, one at discharge from hospital to exclude a complication such as an empyema (infected pleural fluid), one at follow-up about 4 weeks later to ensure complete clearing.

Fig. 4.13.a Added shadowing in the left lower and mid zones, with an air bronchogram within. The left heart border is indistinct, indicating interruption of the normal air/soft tissue interface. Characteristic appearances of lingular consolidation. **b** Lingular consolidation confirmed on the lateral view. Note added density anterior to the oblique fissure (*arrows*).

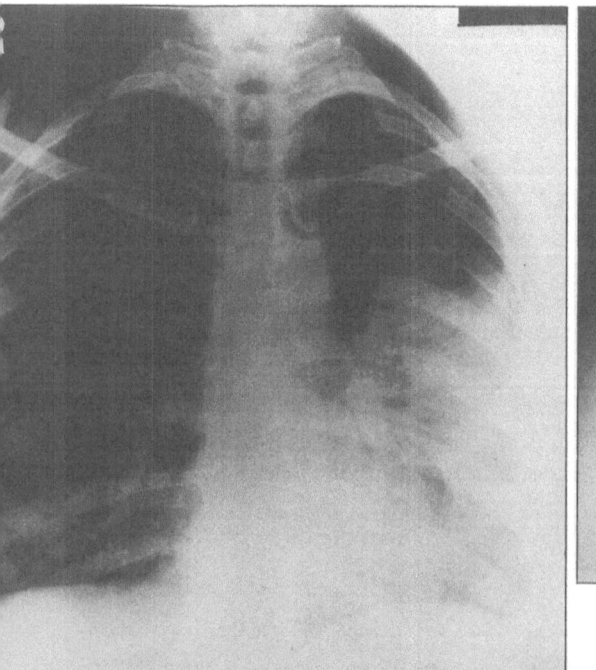
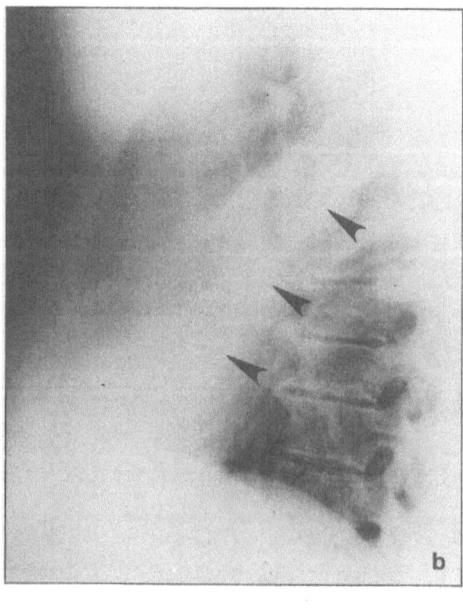

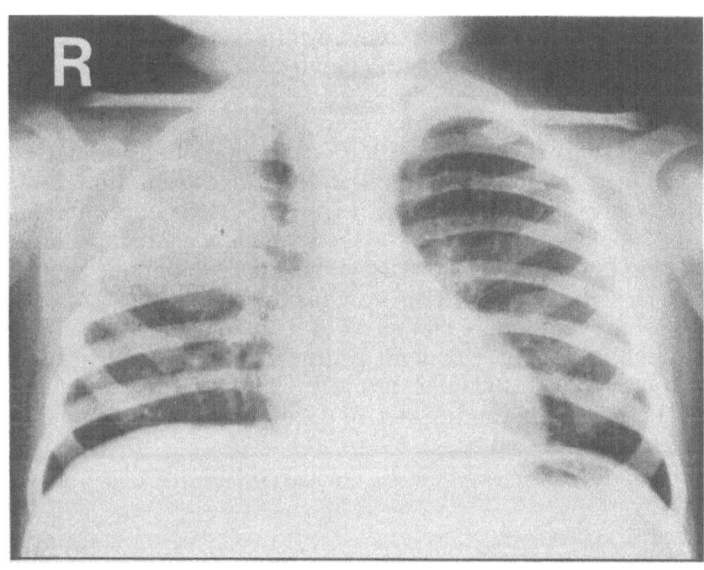

Fig. 4.14. A child with right upper lobe consolidation. See how it abuts the horizontal fissure.

Heart failure

Many CXRs are performed in order to confirm pulmonary oedema. The classic signs of bilateral symmetrical consolidation, obscuring the hilar vessels in a so-called bat's wing distribution, cause little diagnostic difficulty in the correct clinical setting. Such x-rays are usually used as a baseline from which progress can be assessed.

Much more difficult is the detection of the first signs of pulmonary oedema. The CXR may be of great help in differentiating between asthma, chronic bronchitis/emphysema or cardiac failure in the dyspnoeic patient. When the pulmonary venous pressure becomes elevated (from whatever cause, but commonly left ventricular disease or mitral valve problems), the walls of the alveoli in the dependent portions of the lungs become waterlogged, and gas exchange is less efficient than usual. Vasoconstriction in the dependent pulmonary bed causes redistribution to the less congested parts of the lungs, which in the erect position are the upper lobes. This upper lobe blood diversion is a very subjective radiological sign (Fig. 4.15a), and in practice it is only convincing with a baseline normal radiograph for comparison. Some radiologists find that inverting the radiograph is of help; if the upper lobe vessels then look like normal lower lobe vessels, that is taken to be good evidence of redistribution. Another trick is to find an end-on bronchus (that supplying the anterior segment of the upper lobe is often well seen). Normally the bronchus and accompanying vessel are of similar size. If there is upper lobe redistribution, the vessel will appear larger than its accompanying bronchus. To add further confusion to a difficult topic, note that raised pulmonary venous pressure is not the only cause of altered vascular distribution: smoking preferentially affects the lower lobes. When these have become sufficiently damaged, blood will be redistributed to the upper lobes (see Fig. 4.11).

Raised pulmonary venous pressure will also result in interstitial oedema, which in turn causes congestion of the interlobular septa. These show up as fine linear shadows abutting the lung edge (septal lines—Kerley "B" lines after the original description, Fig. 4.15b). They are often associated with a thin lamellar effusion (Fig. 4.15c), which is characteristically seen as a thin layer in the axillary region just above the costophrenic angle. This association provides good evidence of heart failure.

More severe failure can result in large effusions—seemingly commoner on the right. Pulmonary oedema is the final radiological stage of failure. Before becoming obvious with air bronchogram formation, pulmonary oedema may be recognized by causing lack of definition of the pulmonary vasculature, but this is a subtle sign.

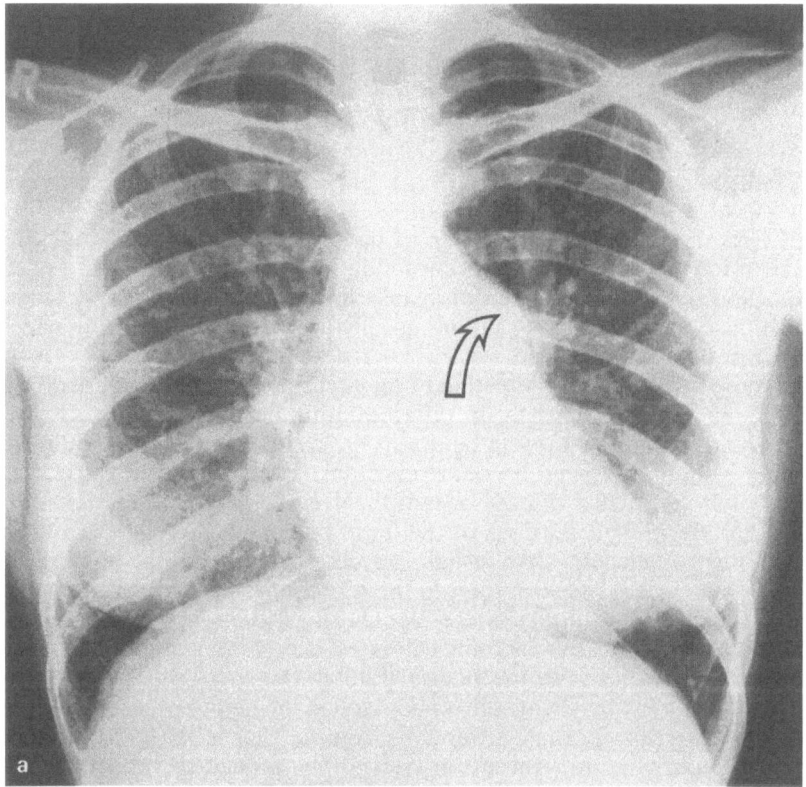

Fig. 4.15.a Raised pulmonary venous pressure in a patient with mitral stenosis. Note the upper-lobe blood diversion and the horizontal septal lines at the lung bases (see **b**). The long-standing pulmonary venous hypertension has led to pulmonary arterial hypertension; hence the large main pulmonary artery (*arrow*). The film is too underexposed to assess the large left atrium (see Fig. 4.6).

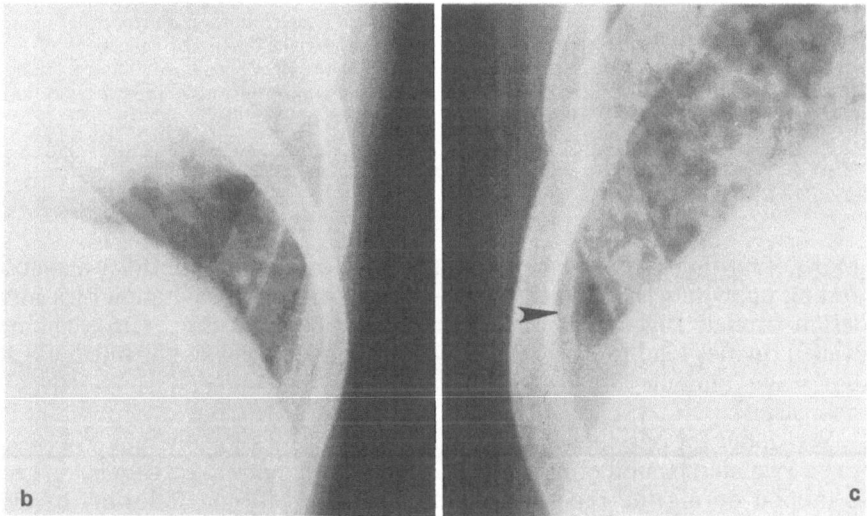

Fig. 4.15.b Enlarged view of the right costophrenic recess in **a** showing linear shadows of fluid in the interlobular septa.

Fig. 4.15.c Enlarged view of the costophrenic recess of another patient with raised pulmonary venous pressure. Septal lines again evident. See also small vertical added density between lung and thoracic cage due to a small lamellar effusion (*arrow*)

Nodules

These can vary in size from pinpoint to large mass lesions. Size, distribution, the presence of cavitation or calcification and other features help the radiologist to suggest likely causes in any given patient. But this is nothing more than an educated guess—inevitable considering the wide range of causes (Scadding 1952). Small nodules must be differentiated from end-on vessels. To clinch the diagnosis a nodule should be identifiable clearly separate from the line of a vessel—not so easy in those diseases where nodular and reticular (linear) shadowing coexist (e.g. many pneumoconioses). Miliary tuberculosis, although rare, is always a potential worry with widespread disseminated nodular shadowing (see Fig. 1.2). An individual miliary focus is probably too small to cast an individual shadow. Superimposition of many foci is required to cause an individual nodule. Thus when miliary tuberculosis is seen on a CXR, the patient will inevitably be very sick. Conversely, it is possible for a patient to die from disseminated tuberculosis with a normal CXR.

A large (5 cm) solitary intrapulmonary opacity will usually turn out to be a tumour (primary or secondary). Sadly, carcinoma of the bronchus is extremely common—every eighth male smoker will succumb to it. Despite this, only rarely can the diagnosis be clinched on radiological grounds (e.g. local bone destruction, phrenic nerve involvement, bone or lung metastases).

Fig. 4.17.a This patient has raised pulmonary venous pressure following a myocardial infarct. The two large well-circumscribed opacities lateral to the right hilum are collections of fluid loculated in the fissures. Note also a lamellar effusion at the right base (*arrow*) and some fluid obscuring the left costophrenic angle. **b** The lateral view confirms the sites of the two collections: **1** in the horizontal fissure, **2** in the superior portion of the oblique film.

▶

More often the CXR will be suggestive of a carcinoma, the final diagnosis resting on cytological studies. Thick-walled (0.5–3 cm) cavitation of a mass lesion strongly suggests a primary bronchial neoplasm (Fig. 4.16). Thinner walled cavities tend to be due to infection (pyogenic abscess or tuberculosis) but some tumours break this rule (notably disseminated squamous cell neoplasms).

Watch out for opacities in the line of fissures. Occasionally they will prove to be loculated pleural effusions (Fig. 4.17). Fluid tends to be trapped in such a fashion during the recovery phase of a large effusion following cardiac failure. The lateral view can be invaluable here—saving unnecessary anxiety and investigation for a nonexistent mass lesion.

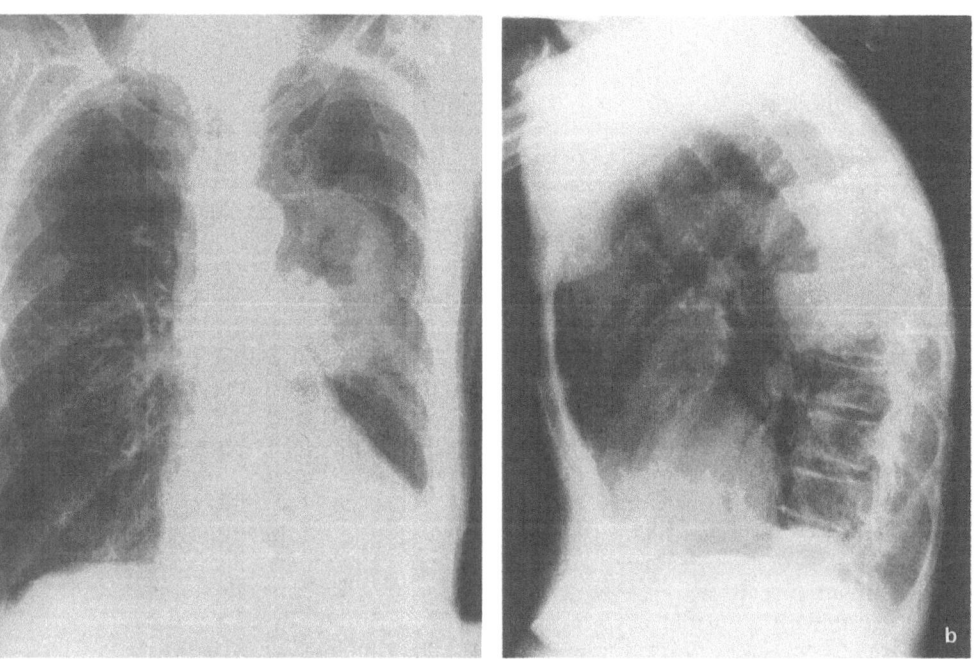

Fig. 4.16. a and **b** Large thick-walled cavity in the apical segment of left lower lobe. Note the air/fluid level. Likely diagnosis: carcinoma of bronchus. Diagnosis clinched by the presence of rib destruction adjacent to the mass. Lesion must be posteriorly situated as the left mediastinal shadow remains sharply defined. This is confirmed on the lateral view (**b**).

Fig. 4.17.a ▶

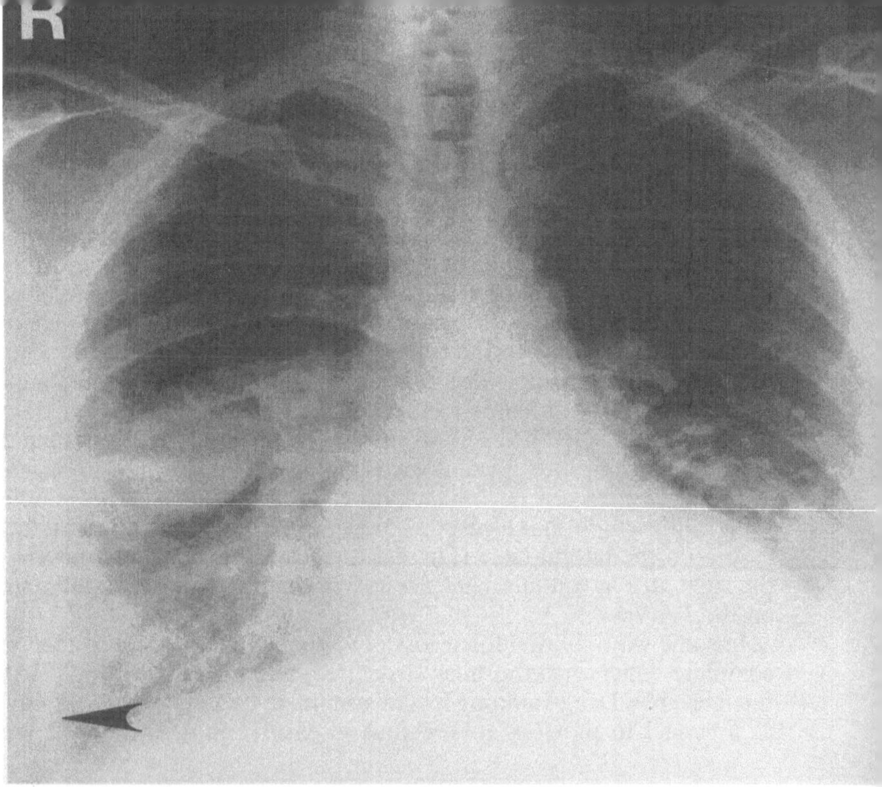

Fig. 4.17.b ▶

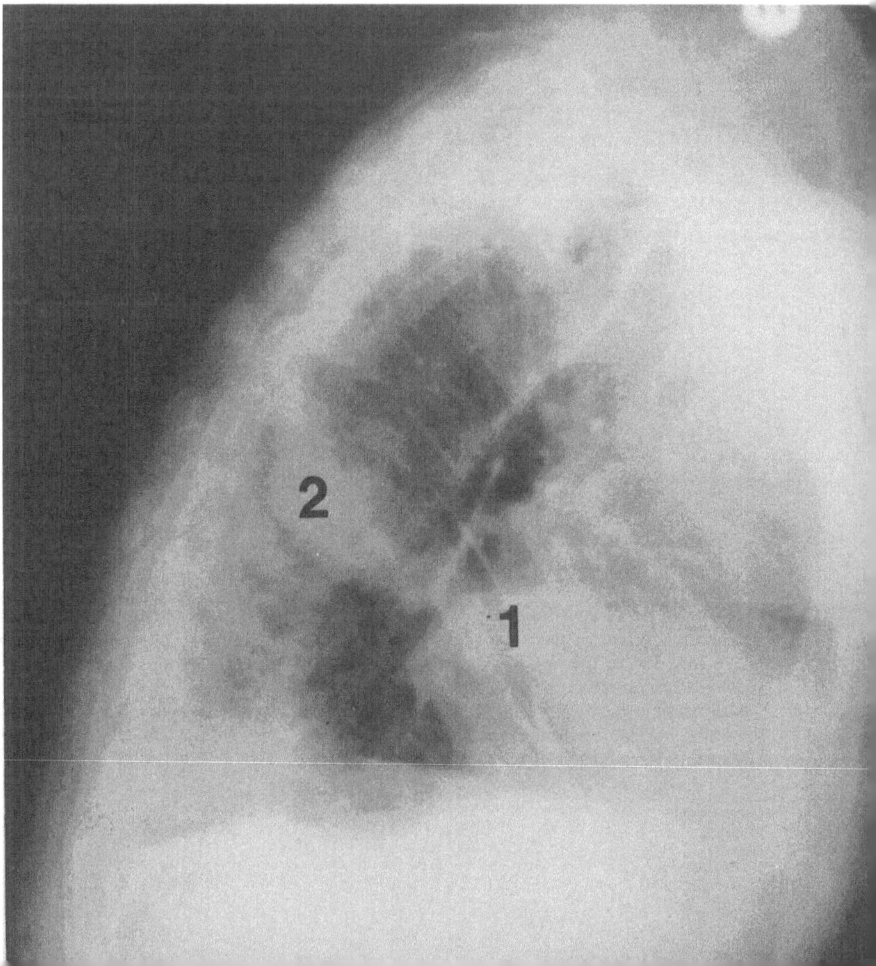

Collapse

Recognition of a collapsed lobe can be difficult. The easiest one to miss is collapse of the left lower lobe, particularly if the film is somewhat under-exposed. Hopefully, the opacity caused by the collapsed lobe will be visible within the left heart border (Fig. 4.18). It will obscure the medial portion of the left dome (normal air/dome interface lost). But even on a pale film there may be clues pointing to the collapse. The left hilum will be low but may not be readily identifiable. The left upper lobe may undergo compensatory emphysema in an attempt to maintain the volume of the left hemithorax. Accordingly, the left hemithorax may then appear more lucent than the right, with the vessels more sparsely distributed.

Similar stories can be told for other lobar collapses. The middle lobe is rather different in that it just collapses down to a wedge abutting the oblique fissure on the lateral view (Fig. 4.19). Again this opaque structure abutting the right atrium will interrupt the normal sharp (air/heart) right heart border on the PA view.

In some ways, partial lobar loss of volume may be easier to recognize than complete collapse as the hilar structures, although low or high, will still be recognizable. Long-standing loss of volume of an upper lobe is still often seen as a sequel to previous tuberculous disease (Fig. 4.20). The hilum on the

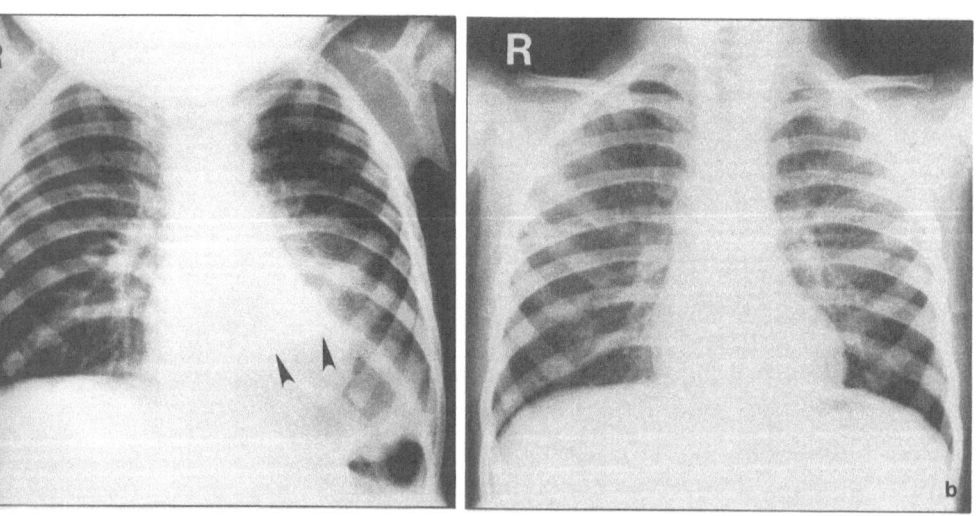

Fig. 4.18.a Left lower-lobe collapse in a child who had aspirated a peanut. Increased opacity within the left heart border with loss of the normal sharp lung/left dome interface (*arrows*). Left hilum low due to the lower lobe loss of volume. Compare with **b** The same child when fully recovered. Normal appearances.

Remember that foreign bodies more usually pass into the right main bronchus (it is more vertical). Furthermore, they may cause a ball-valve obstruction with overinflation rather than collapse.

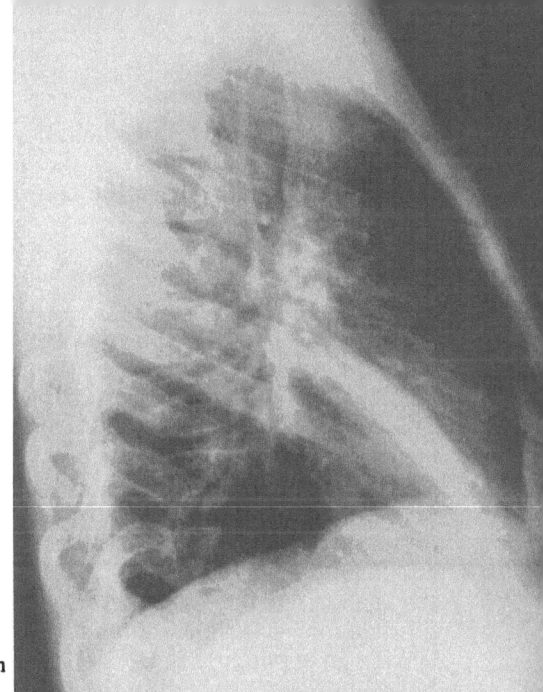

Fig. 4.19. Lateral view of a child with middle-lobe collapse. See how the horizontal fissure has approximated to the oblique fissure to form a band shadow—the airless middle lobe.

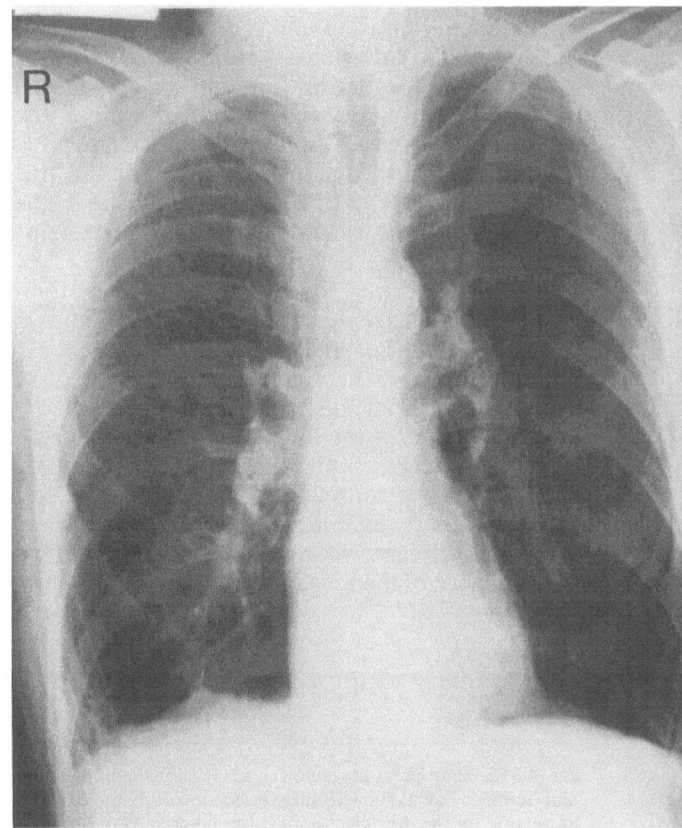

Fig. 4.20. Left hilar elevation in this elderly patient. This is due to loss of volume of the upper lobe following previous tuberculosis. There is not much in the way of calcification in the upper lobe which would make the diagnosis easier. Note low flat domes indicating some emphysema.

affected side will be elevated and, if on the right, the horizontal fissure will be bowed upwards in characteristic fashion. Scattered calcification in the shrunken lobe will confirm the diagnosis.

Pleural effusion

Nearly all CXRs are obtained in the erect position. Accordingly, *free* pleural fluid will gravitate to abut the diaphragm. Luckily for radiologists, a layer of such fluid usually tracks up in the pleural space between lung and chest wall. This collection of fluid blunts the costophrenic angle (see Fig. 4.17a) and, as it increases in volume, it may be seen end on as a thick vertical opaque band in the axillary region. Of course, there is nothing magical about the axillary region, and there will be a similar layer of free fluid in the anterior and posterior portions of the hemithorax; but these may not be thick enough to attenuate the x-ray beam noticeably. The normal sharp air/dome interface of the appropriate hemithorax is usually obscured, but in the erect position it is possible for *mobile* pleural fluid to layer out between the dome and the lung, leaving an apparently sharp air/"dome" margin. A decubitus film (see Chap. 5, "*Plain films*"), whereby the fluid is shifted into the axillary region, will identify such *subpulmonary effusions* (Fig. 4.21). Apart from catches like the subpulmonary effusion and the loculated (fissure) effusion (see "*Nodules*"), simple mobile effusions, say due to cardiac failure, should be easily recognized. Clues as to aetiology (septal lines in cardiac failure) may be present. Not so easy are effusions of a more viscous nature (e.g. pus in an empyema), or those where the fluid is trapped by pleural adhesions. These can cause bizarre shadows, but on either the PA or lateral CXR the peripheral nature of the lesion should be evident. In cases of doubt, an oblique tangential view of the lesion might help—one of the few situations where an oblique view might be justified. Fluoroscopy will be even more reliable in localizing the lesion. Sometimes there will be a need to decide whether a localized pleural lesion is due to fluid or tumour: ultrasound should reveal an echo-free pattern if fluid, and may help in localization before aspiration.

One other problem is the effusion so large as to fill the hemithorax with fluid and render it totally opaque. This will usually be due to a malignancy. Here the mediastinum may get pushed by the fluid and ultimately begin to compromise the contralateral normal lung. Often there is some collapse of the lung underlying a large effusion, so that mediastinal displacement is not evident. This cause of an opaque hemithorax must be distinguished from a total collapse of the lung, which will pull the mediastinum towards the opaque

⟶

Fig. 4.21.a Semi-erect portable AP CXR showing poor definition at the left base. **b** Decubitus film (left side down) showing huge collection of fluid in left pleural space (*arrows*). This was hard to identify on the AP film where it has layered posteriorly and in the subpulmonary space.

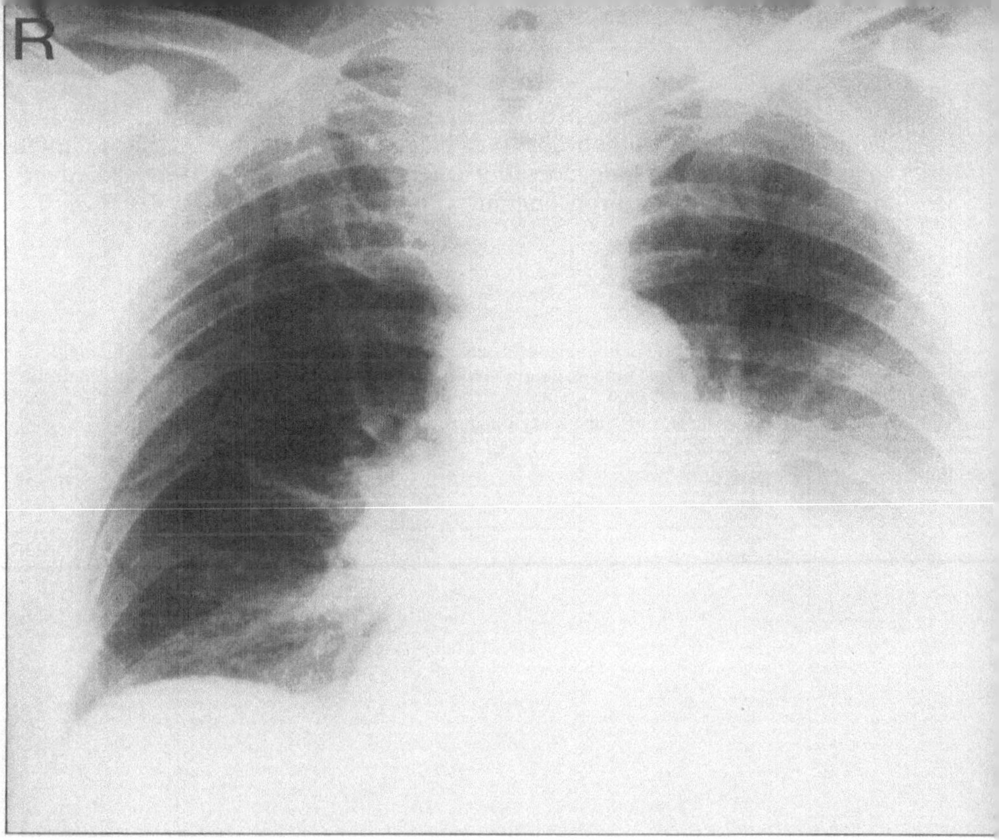

Fig. 4.21.a ▲

Fig. 4.21.b ▼

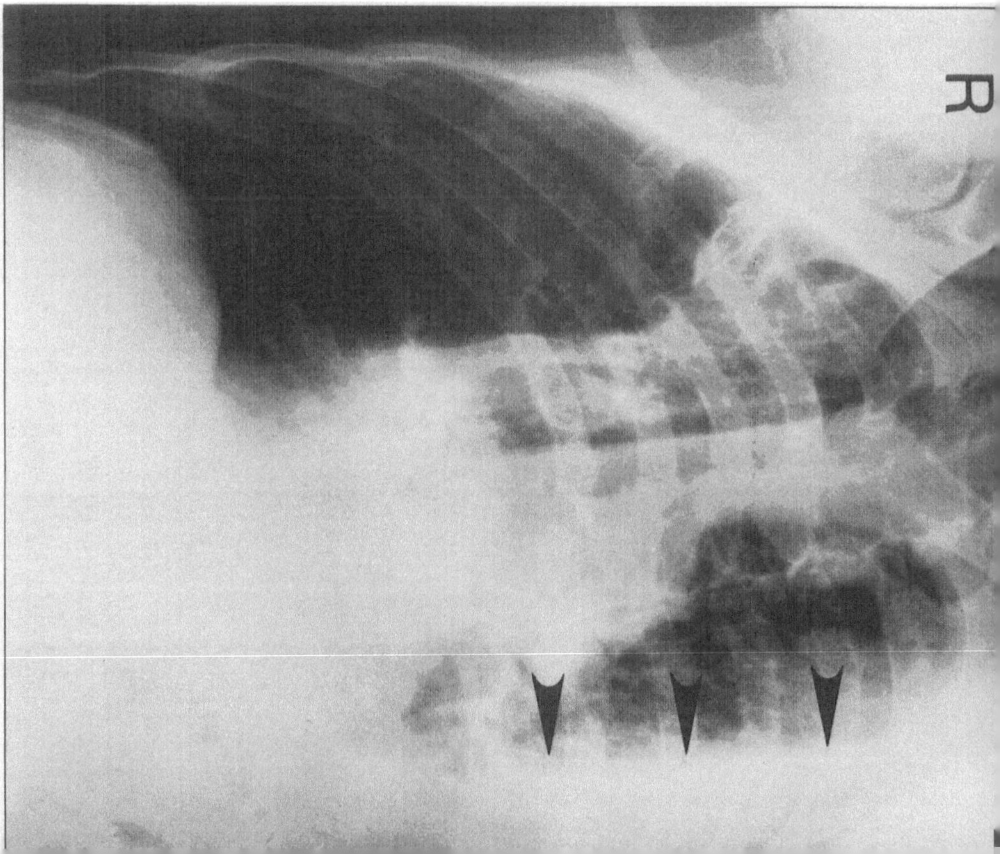

hemithorax. The hypothetically possible opaque hemithorax due to total consolidation of one lung does not often occur in practice—it should be recognizable by the air bronchogram within.

References

Fraser RG, Paré JAP (1977) Diagnosis of diseases of the chest, 2nd edn. Saunders, Philadelphia
Scadding JG (1952) Chronic lung disease with diffuse nodular or reticular radiographic shadows. Tubercle 33:352
Simon G (1971) Principles of chest x-ray diagnosis, 3rd edn. Butterworths, London

5. The Abdomen

Plain films

Most patients admitted with an "acute abdomen" will have erect and supine x-ray films. These usually provide helpful clues about what is going on, confirming or refuting the provisional clinical diagnoses made by the general practitioner or casualty officer. The *supine* film is the standard examination, and should cover everything in the abdomen from diaphragm to pubis. The *erect* film is done to look for *fluid levels* in the bowel, and for free intraperitoneal gas below the diaphragm (so it must include that muscle!). Note that the essential prerequisite in this projection is for the x-ray beam to be *horizontal*, parallel to fluid/solid interfaces. Patients may well be too ill to stand upright, even for a minute, but that is never a reason for omitting this useful projection. The patient can always be turned on his side, obtaining an AP projection with a horizontal x-ray beam. This is the "lateral decubitus" position in radiography parlance. It would have been better if the supine and erect films had been christened vertical and horizontal x-ray beam films. It is now too late to change this usage, but be sure you understand what is really important about these positionings: the direction of the x-ray beam, not the patient's posture.

Much of what goes amiss in the upper abdomen has repercussions above the diaphragm; or a primary lesion which is above the diaphragm (e.g. lower lobe pneumonia) may present with abdominal symptoms. For these reasons a *chest film* is very often a helpful third routine radiograph. The assessment of any patient with undiagnosed acute abdominal pain cannot be considered complete without it.

Gut obstruction

The bowel is dilated (gas distended) down to the site of obstruction, and empty of gas beyond. This is a key fact for siting the level of hold-up, and also for deciding whether obstruction is present at all. If there is generalized distension of small *and* large bowel, then *paralytic ileus* is a more likely diagnosis than obstruction (a very low obstruction, e.g. in the rectum, is not commonly accompanied by secondary small-bowel dilatation).

How to decide this important matter, whether the dilated loops are small or large bowel or both? The rules (Table 5.1) are simple enough, but their interpretation is not. Do not be taken in by the notion that "plain films" must be about something humdrum and straightforward, by contrast with complex high-falutin matters like arteriograms. Plain-film interpretation of the acute abdomen is difficult, but rewarding for patient and doctor. It sorts out the men from the boys—here, the thoughtful from the lackadaisical. Try to emerge with a definite conclusion of your own: *does* the patient suffer from obstruction, and if so *where*? If doubts remain, follow-up films 24 h later may help to resolve them.

The clinical circumstances are of course a very helpful and legitimate clue, which you should have by your side in reading these films. *Small-bowel obstruction* is an acute presentation with pain and vomiting over hours rather than days. *Large-bowel obstruction* is of insidious onset, often extending over days or weeks of slowly increasing discomfort and girth. *Ileus* is characteristically a postoperative event, with a large, silent abdomen. The patient cannot pass flatus, even though the rectum is distended with gas.

Table 5.1 Gas patterns to distinguish between small- and large-bowel dilatation

	Site in the abdomen	Gas pattern
Small bowel	Central	Valvulae conniventes present in upper gut: ring-like folds encircling the lumen — imagine a coilspring forming the innermost lining of the bowel (Fig. 5.1).
Large bowel	Peripheral	Haustra indent *one* aspect of the colon: incomplete impressions tethering part of the wall — imagine a short length of Sellotape stuck circularly on one-half of the bowel circumference (Fig. 5.2).

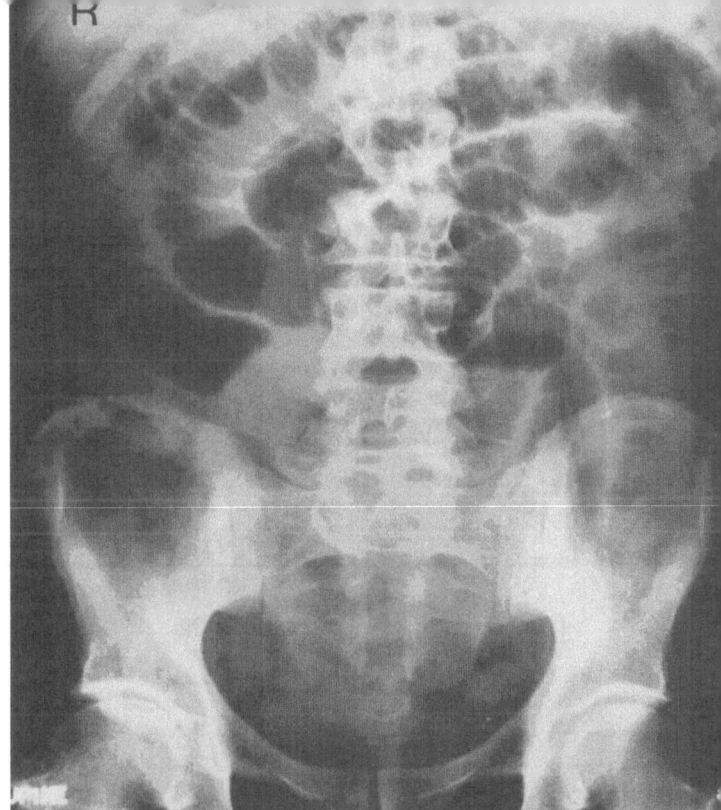

Fig. 5.1.a On this supine film of the abdomen several dilated, gas-distended small-bowel loops are seen. They are centrally placed in the abdomen, and have a coilspring-like pattern on their insides—the valvulae conniventes. There is no gas distal to these loops—this patient has small-bowel obstruction.
b Because of obstruction, there is severe stasis of small bowel contents, separated out on this erect film into gas/fluid interfaces—so-called fluid levels. The end of the gastric aspiration tube has a metal tip—note that the stomach is marked by a further fluid level beneath the left hemi-diaphragm.

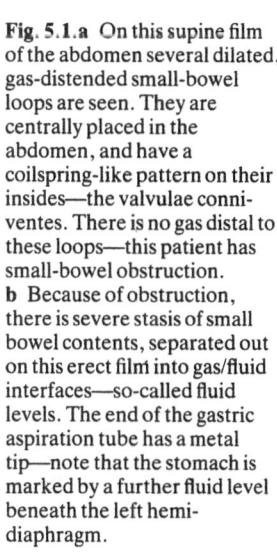

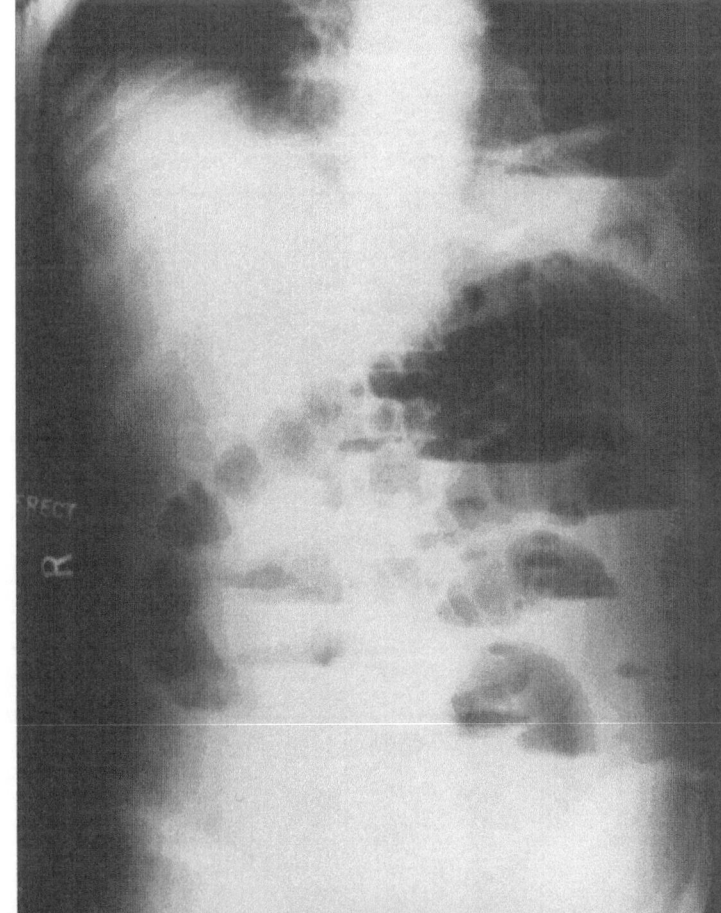

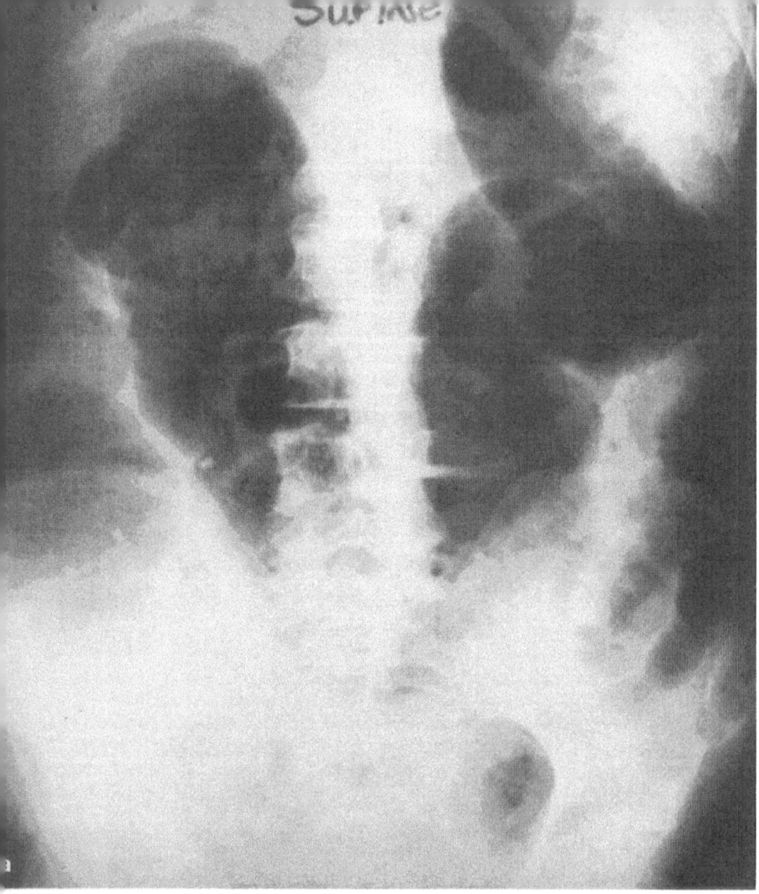

Fig. 5.2.a This patient also has gaseous distension of bowel, but the loops are larger, more peripheral, and indented for part of their diameter by extrinsic haustra.

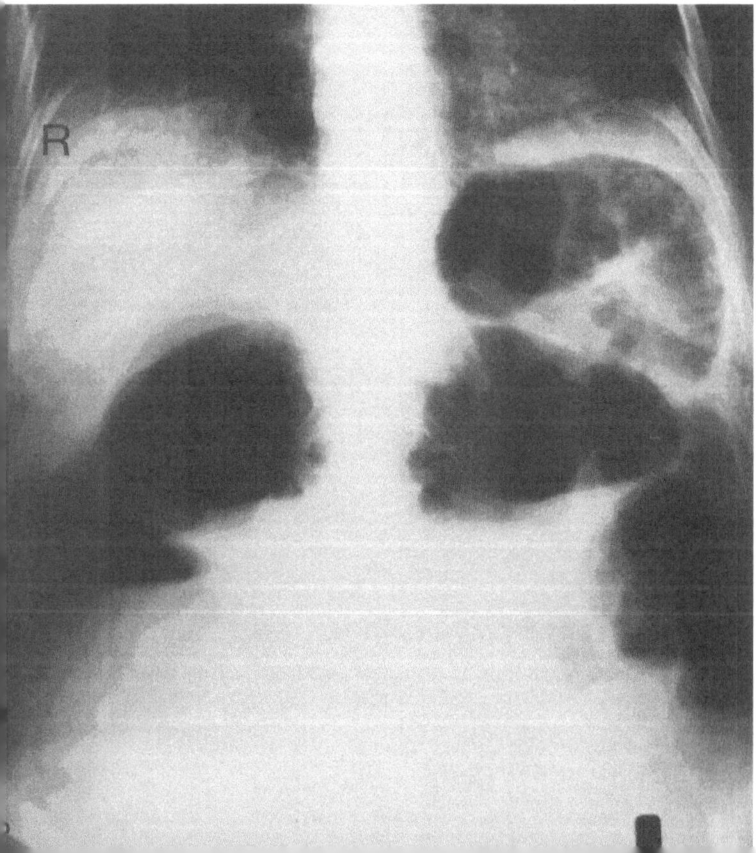

Fig. 5.2.b The erect film again shows fluid levels in dilated large gut loops, with no gas in the distal colon. This is large-bowel obstruction.

Perforation

Sudden pain with a rigid abdomen: you must have a horizontal beam (e.g. erect) film including the diaphragm here to look for peritoneal gas (Fig. 5.3). Careful—the gas must be intraperitoneal to make this diagnosis, not just in the stomach immediately below the left hemidiaphragm, or in a hepatic flexure interposed between liver and right hemidiaphragm (Fig. 5.4).

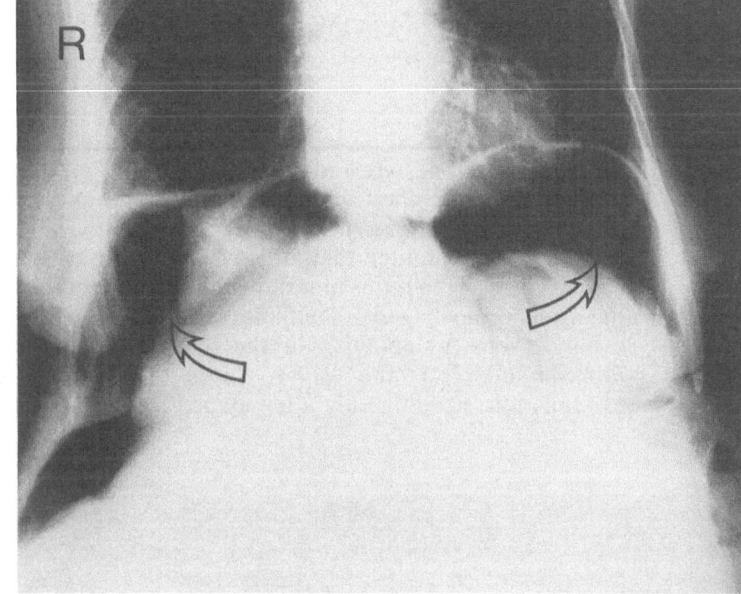

Fig. 5.3. Erect film showing large gas collections beneath each hemidiaphragm (*arrows*). This is free intraperitoneal gas following perforation of the bowel (sigmoid diverticulitis). Note how the liver beneath the right hemidiaphragm and the large bowel beneath the left hemidiaphragm have been made visible by the intra-peritoneal gas.

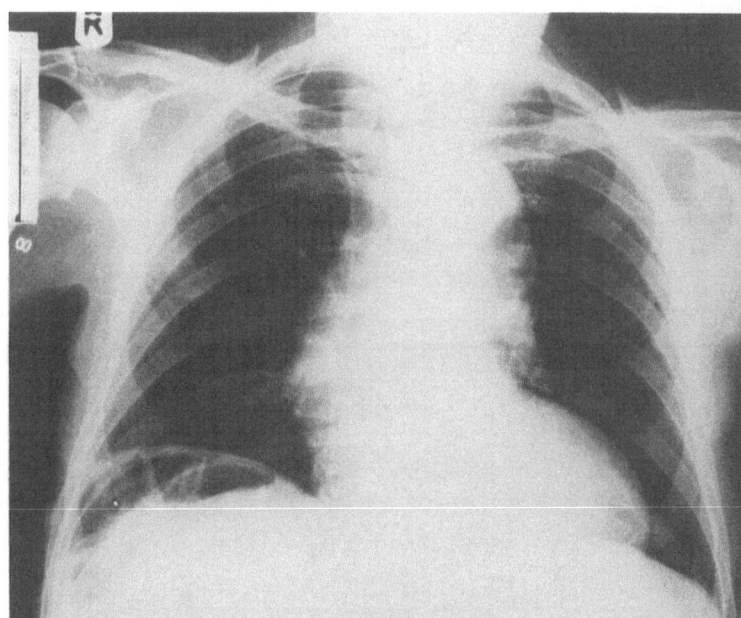

Fig. 5.4. The gas shadows beneath the right hemi-diaphragm in this patient are clearly contained in some tubular structure, with haustra running across it. This is a loop of colon interposed between the liver and right hemi-diaphragm—a normal variant.

Acute cholecystitis

Most gallstones are not radio-opaque. The normal plain film therefore does nothing to invalidate this diagnosis. An immediate *ultrasound scan* can be helpful here: it may show gallstones, and a distended, oedematous gallbladder. But an immediate *radionuclide scan* is the most useful step. A labelled agent excreted by the hepatocyte is injected. The characteristic image in this disease shows the liver at work, the common bile duct full of activity, and yet no sign of gallbladder activity. The examination has great specificity, i.e. a normal finding, with activity in the gallbladder, excludes acute cholecystitis from the differential diagnosis.

Ureteric colic

Most kidney stones are radio-opaque. There are important exceptions: uric acid or matrix stones, blood clot and necrotic papillae are examples of nonopaque plugs that may obstruct a ureter. The normal plain film is therefore no guarantee that all is well with the patient suspected of ureteric colic. Worse, even if this film shows an opaque something in the line of one of the ureters, the diagnosis is still not secure. Is it an unimportant concretion in a pelvic vein (phlebolith), or the real thing? The emergency *intravenous urogram* (IVU) is the way to settle the question: this can be a short examination, needing only a few films (Fig. 3.5).

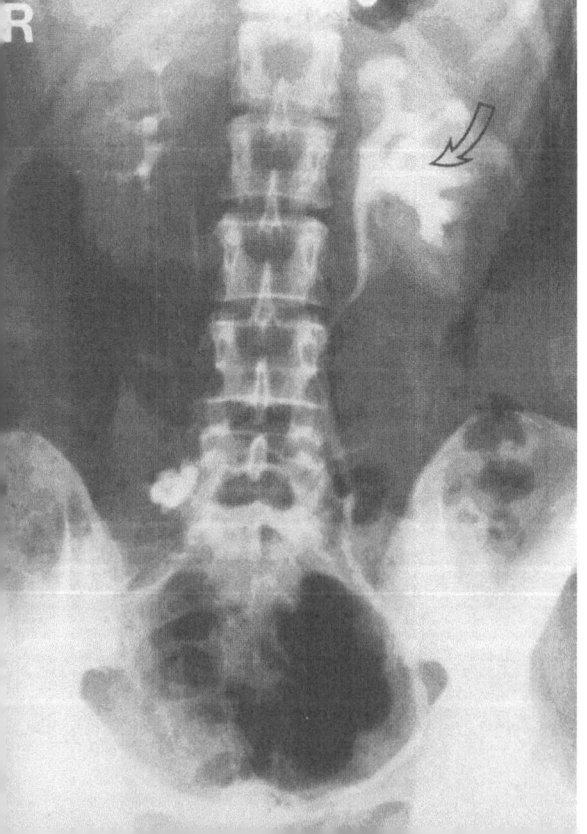

Fig. 5.5. This patient has left ureteric colic. On her IVU the right kidney is normal, but the whole of the left upper urinary tract is distended down to a small stone in her left ureter (hidden by the surrounding contrast medium in the ureter on this film). Acute obstruction by this stone has been severe enough to rupture the kidney—note the tell-tale sliver of opacified urine escaping into the renal sinus alongside the renal pelvis (*arrow*). Such tears will heal spontaneously once the obstructing stone has been passed or removed.

Why an emergency IVU when most ureteric stones do not need urgent surgery? There are two reasons. There may be indecision about an important alternative diagnosis calling for action, e.g. right ureteric colic versus appendicitis. Secondly, a positive diagnosis has real value for determining the future course of action. If a patient has a ureteric stone, he will need full metabolic investigation, and the rest of his life may be coloured by what is found. Contrast this diagnostic certainty with the cloud of vague worry if a "cold" IVU is done 3 weeks later and is then normal. Did he or did he not have a ureteric stone, since passed? Does he need further investigation?

The ureteric-colic IVU makes or breaks the diagnosis: if it is normal the patient cannot have upper urinary tract obstruction. Note that the IVU is therefore very reliable about *acute* obstruction. This does not apply to *chronic* obstruction.

Ultrasound

Making radar or echo maps of the human body is harmless and painless. A pencil beam of ultrasound is shone into the patient, and the reflected echoes are recorded. Such images depend on the acoustic elasticity of tissues, a very different matter to the x-ray absorption characteristics determining radiographs. Ultrasound images are most commonly displayed as cross-sectional maps along transverse or longitudinal (parasagittal) planes. It is also possible to obtain a continuous, moving image of such a plane: "real-time" ultrasound. In this way the fetus can be watched moving in utero—a magical sight.

Obstetrics is the historical starting point of medical ultrasound. Since the fertilized ovum can be monitored from a few weeks old, normal and abnormal pregnancies can be followed step by step. The fetus lies in a bag of fluid—an excellent medium for transmitting ultrasound. Gas and bone will not transmit ultrasound at diagnostic frequencies. Overlying bowel gas or ribs are therefore awkward barriers to examining abdominal organs. Fat patients also make for poor ultrasound images (but for good CT ones!).

Because of the different echo characteristics of fluid and solid tissues, ultrasound is good at answering questions like: "Is this lump in the kidney an unimportant cyst or a probable tumour?" or: "Does this alcoholic have a pancreatic pseudocyst, or a pancreatic tumour?" Obstetric, gynaecological, kidney, pancreas and liver problems are the most frequent indications for abdominal ultrasound (see "*Jaundice*" below).

Gallstones make up fine hunting country for ultrasound (Fig. 5.6). Remember we are here concerned with the patient suffering from chronic symptoms which might be because of gallstones—the patient with acute cholecystitis (see above) needs quite different investigative attention. Ultrasound is taking over the reins from an older gallstone hunt: the oral cholecystogram, an x-ray technique where a contrast medium is absorbed and excreted by the patient in order to opacify the gallbladder (Fig. 5.7). This is a useless test in jaundice!

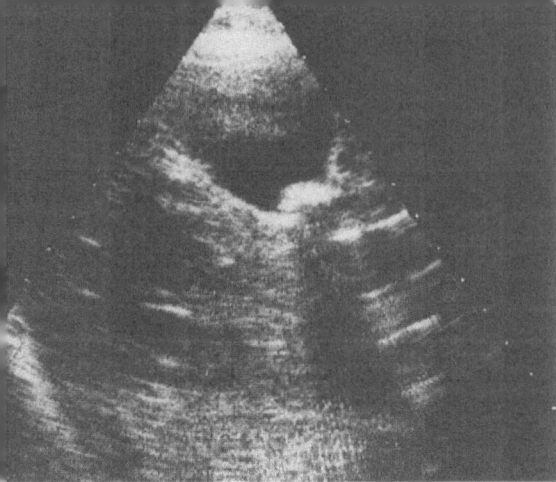

Fig. 5.6. Longitudinal ultrasound scan of the liver—the black, echo-free bag is the gall-bladder. In its bottom sits a small, reflecting (*white*) gallstone, with an acoustic corridor (*black*) behind it, where it stops the transmission of sound waves.

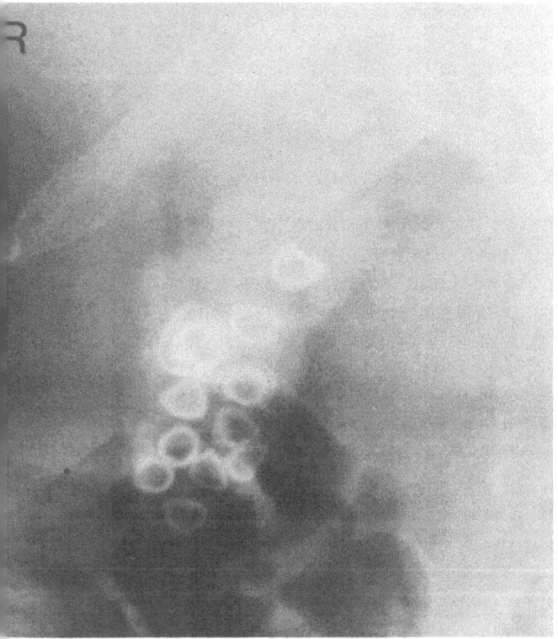

Fig.5.7.a A gallbladder containing multiple, faceted gallstones. The gallbladder has been faintly outlined because the patient is excreting a biliary contrast medium, taken by mouth. A plain film is very helpful when gallstones are radio-opaque like this, but most are not.
b Another patient having an oral cholecysto-gram, opacifying her gallbladder. There are ten small radiolucent gallstones surrounding one larger central radiolucent stone. They are only made visible against the contrast medium in the gallbladder— a characteristic of most gallstones. stones.

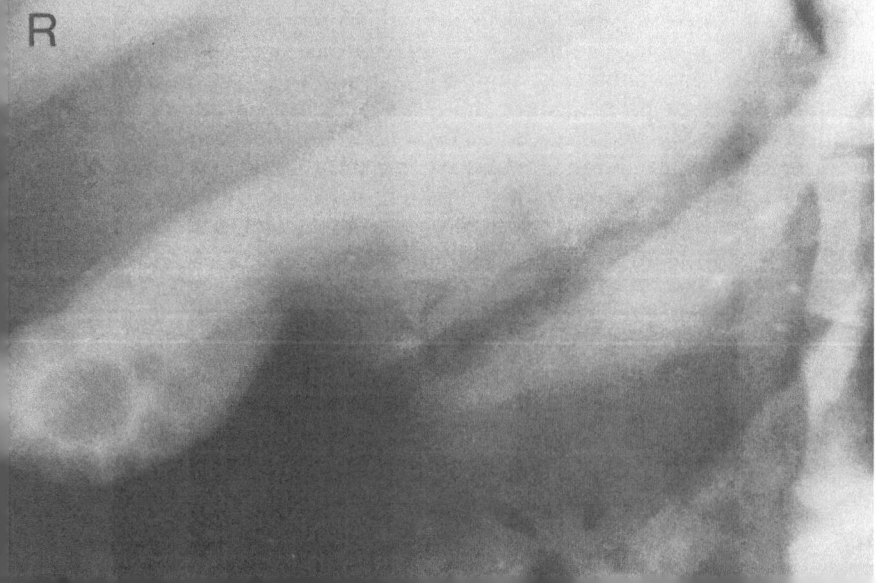

Ultrasound and CT are techniques using two-dimensional, sectional anatomy displays. A number of such sections may be required in order to build up a good composite picture of the organ under study. It is as if you are finding out about a birthday cake only through examining each slice in turn. A radiograph will show you the cake whole, but in all likelihood overlayed by much unwanted information: the other food on the table, the guests' feet below it, their hands reaching out above, etc.

Jaundice

All hospital medicine used to be divided into two parts. "Are you medical or surgical?" was asked of patients, diseases and students in the same sort of way as allegiance to Oxford or Cambridge for the Boat Race. It was inadvisable even to attempt diagnosis if one was in the wrong camp: "Oh it's not medical/surgical" was sufficient dismissal. Those days are largely past, but for the jaundiced patient the distinction remains of great importance. Dark urine and pale stools have long been recognized as a surgical problem, pointing to biliary tree obstruction. A battery of ever more refined biochemical tests has been added to help differentiate prehepatic and hepatocellular (medical) from posthepatic (surgical) jaundice. The clinical background together with these tests may well point to a clear answer, but clinical doubt is common. Most of the time we have to ask, "Could this be surgically correctable jaundice, for instance a stone in the common bile duct?" The first step towards an answer is a good ultrasound scan. Dilated intrahepatic bile ducts will be seen in biliary obstruction. We have to use a decision tree here—an example of trial-and-error scientific investigation (Fig. 5.8).

The aim is to spread a safety net beneath the patient so that he does not drop into a dangerous cul-de-sac of misdiagnosis. The ultrasound scan (about 80%–90% accurate) might fail to show the patient's dilated bile ducts during the early days or even weeks of the illness. Very well, we will do a radionuclide scan in this group. Note that this sort of scheme is quite different from the blunderbuss "it's-so-important-that-we-must-do-every-test-in-sight" approach. It is also easy to update a decision tree as new knowledge accrues.

The *percutaneous cholangiogram* involves passing a very fine needle into the liver under local anaesthesia. It sounds unattractive for the patient, but is in fact remarkably well tolerated, and also safe. Having a precise preoperative diagnosis and map of what will be found can be most helpful at surgery (Fig. 5.9).

Barium meal

The patient swallows an insoluble suspension of barium sulphate, which will outline the digestive tract on fluoroscopy. It would be a highly toxic substance if given parenterally, but is wholly innocuous as an unabsorbable intestinal passenger. The patient has to fast for several hours before, in order to clear

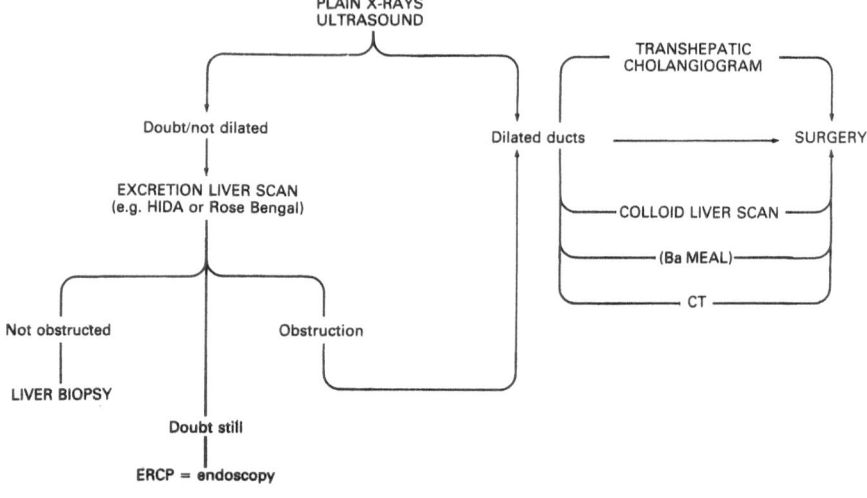

Fig. 5.8. Diagnostic pathway for jaundice.

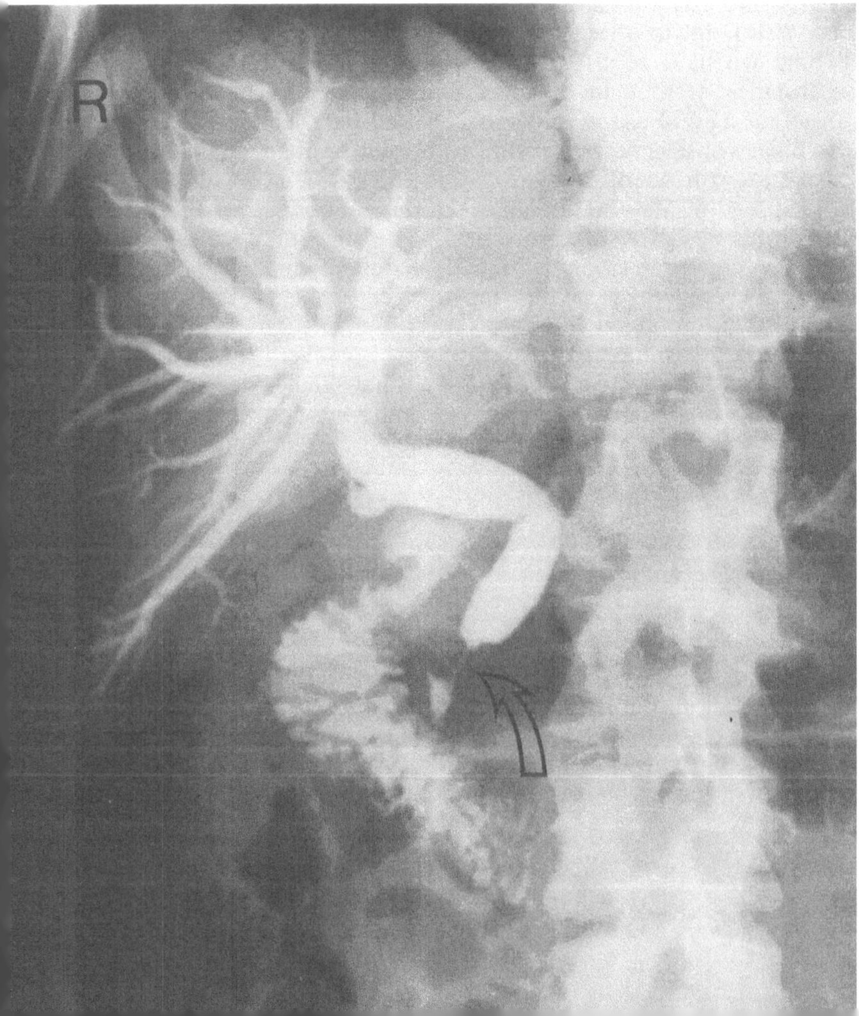

◀ **Fig. 5.9**

the upper gastrointestinal tract of the food residues which would obscure the best views of its lining.

The barium meal is good at answering questions like "Does this patient have an oesophageal stricture/gastric or duodenal ulcer/gastric carcinoma?" It is poor at finding lesions like pancreatic carcinoma, gastric erosions, or gastritis. A simple decision rule for the appropriate barium meal has recently been put forward, well supported by facts (Lancet editorial 1980). Consider a barium meal in a patient with abdominal pain only if (1) he is over 50 years old; or (2) there is a story of a previous peptic ulcer; or (3) pain occurs within an hour of eating; or (4) pain is relieved by food or milk. Note that repeated examinations of a duodenal ulcer are worthless. Active ulceration cannot be distinguished from chronic scarring.

There is now considerable debate about whether it is *useful* to have an accurate diagnosis for the indigestion suffered by a patient under 50 years. Whether the cause is gastritis or a duodenal ulcer, treatment (the indigestion pills or medicine in favour at the time) will be dictated by the symptoms, not the disease. More serious alternative causes of indigestion are uncommon below 50. This is not a generally accepted view by any means. But you should know that there need not be an automatic reflex to write "barium meal please" each time a 40 year old with indigestion consults you. An instructive experiment happened perforce in an English country town quite recently. There was a long waiting list for barium meals. Worse, rebuilding of the x-ray department meant that the service had to be curtailed rather than expanded for 3 months. The local doctors were warned of this. When the x-ray department re-opened ready to fire on all cylinders, the 6 months' large backlog was reviewed, and each doctor was asked which patients still needed barium meals because of continuing symptoms. The answer was about 5%. In short, most patients with indigestion get better, with or without diagnosis.

Endoscopy of the upper gastrointestinal tract is an investigation of rather greater accuracy, but also greater discomfort. It will sometimes follow after the barium meal, e.g. to biopsy a gastric ulcer. It will sometimes make barium studies superfluous, e.g. in the patient with a haematemesis, where they are second best.

Barium enema

Carcinoma of the colon is one of the few cancers curable by surgery. It is also very common, and can present in nonspecific ways, for instance as unexplained tiredness secondary to anaemia. For these reasons radiologists are very concerned to find such tumours accurately at an early stage. This needs a

Fig. 5.9. Transhepatic percutaneous cholangiogram. A very fine needle has been passed into the liver, and contrast medium injected into the dilated biliary tree. The common bile duct is very considerably dilated, obstructed by a carcinoma near its lower end (*arrow*). A little contrast medium has moved through into the duodenum.

meticulous barium enema, including careful wash-out of the bowel before-hand. It is very much a special examination, an ordeal for the patient and a painstaking exercise for the radiologist. Do not request it lightheartedly in the manner of "Abdominal cramps, Mrs Fartingbrass? We'd better just have a barium enema".

The good barium enema will outline small structures such as polyps in the colon (Fig. 5.10). Surgeon and radiologist must then discuss proper manage-ment of this possibly precancerous lesion. Ulcerative colitis and colonic Crohn's disease are examples of inflammatory diseases where the barium enema plays a vital part in diagnosis and monitoring progress. Another example is shown in Fig. 5.11.

The most important message about the barium enema has been left to this last paragraph. A patient with blood in his stools needs a *rectal examination* and *sigmoidoscopy*. Reach for the x-ray request form if these examinations are normal or show piles (the patient may still have a carcinoma!).

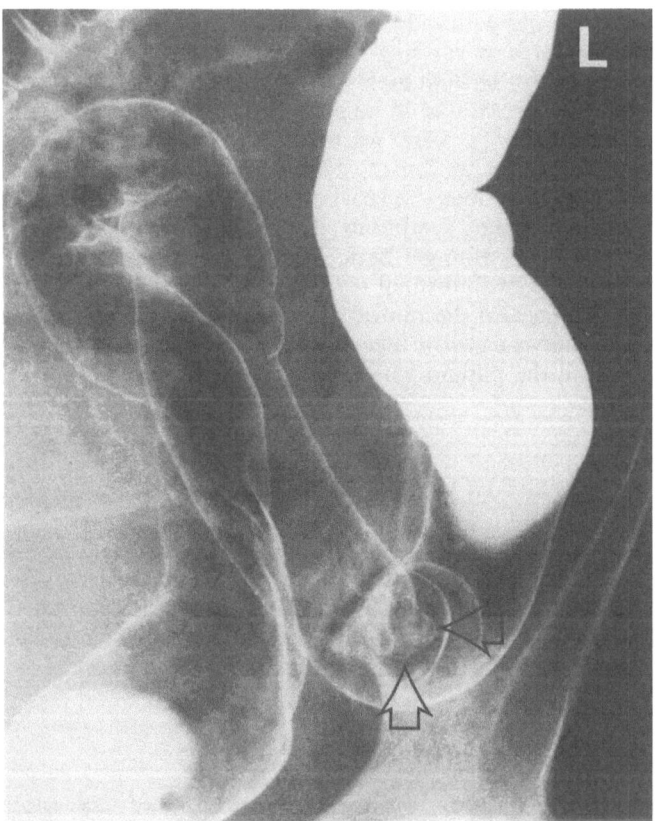

Fig. 5.10. A polyp is shown at the junction of the descending and sigmoid colon, outlined by barium and air on this barium enema (*arrows*).

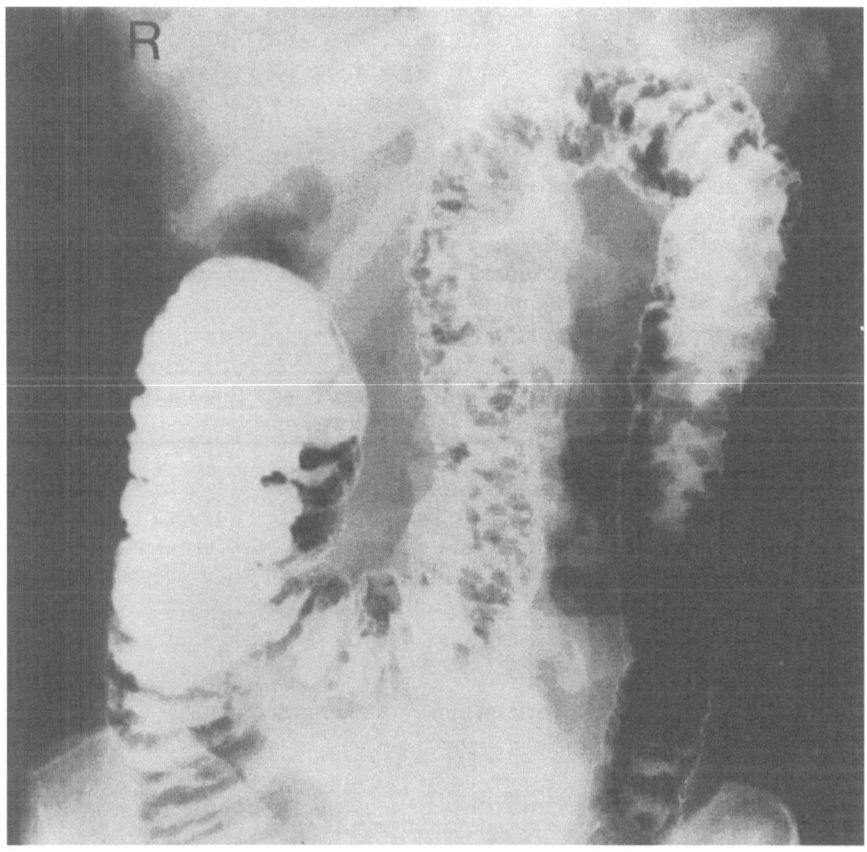

Fig. 5.11. Barium and air on this enema outline a grossly abnormal colonic wall. The interior of the large gut is very irregular, and multiple small ragged nodules and plaques project into the lumen. This is the picture of an extensive colitis—the features in this case point to the complex known as pseudomembranous colitis.

Intravenous urogram (IVU)

The most important message comes first here. It is more or less the same as for the barium enema. The adult patient with haematuria needs a *cystoscopy* to find his bladder tumour, not an IVU (which will probably miss it).

The IVU needs the intravenous injection of a large amount of an organic acid, bearing iodine atoms locked into its structure. This contrast medium is so called because the iodine opacifies the urinary tract for the radiographs as it is excreted (by glomerular filtration). If you think of it as radiopaque inulin, you will not go wrong in interpreting what you see on the films. First, the contrast medium in the glomerular filtrate lights up the whole kidney, the *nephrogram* (see Fig. 5.5). A few minutes later, calices, ureters and bladder will be shown by the contrast-laden urine.

Details of IVU diagnosis are beyond the scope of this book. The majority of patients suspected of nephrological or urological disorders will have an IVU. You should therefore know something of the *limitations* of the examination.

1) It is essentially a test of the *structural* integrity of the urinary tract. Inferences about renal function and urinary transport can often be drawn. However, the IVU is *not* a test of divided or overall renal function.

Plasma creatinine or urea are good overall renal function tests, the *radionuclide renogram* or *scintigram* the best divided function study, weighing one kidney's performance against the other's.

2) The IVU does not provide anything like a complete assessment of the lower urinary tract (bladder and urethra). Remember particularly the bladder tumour diagnosis mentioned in the first paragraph of this section. The IVU can never exclude this lesion, so be careful not to mismanage patients on this account.

3) Severe contrast medium "reactions" are rare, life-threatening hazards of these examinations. Any patient who has suffered such a reaction should only have further parenteral contrast medium studies with great caution. The nature of the reactions is still not understood, but they are certainly not "iodine sensitivity" phenomena. To put the hazard into perspective, the risks of death are very roughly:

IVU	1 in 40 000
Intravenous cholangiogram or gastrointestinal endoscopy	1 in 4 000
Death from any cause in the next year at aet. 40	1 in 400

Envoy

These sections have touched on only a few matters of radiological interest in the abdomen. If you have a puzzle over any patient, or do not know what test to ask for next, there is a simple rule: talk to your radiologists, and encourage them to talk to you.

Reference

Lancet editorial (1980) Sense and sensitivity about the barium meal. Lancet i: 1171–1172

6.   The Skull

The brain is insufficiently dense to be visualized by ordinary radiography, but something can be learnt about the intracranial structures from the appearance of the surrounding bone.

The skull is not easy to examine radiographically due to superimposition on plain films of the complex images of the cranial and facial structures, the upper and lower jaws and the teeth. This makes the interpretation of these images difficult unless one has available a series of standard radiographic projections taken in different planes. These projections are used internationally, so wherever you practise medicine (within reason!) they should appear to you as old friends and give you comfort in your anxiety.

Skull projections

Lateral projection

This projection is used to assess the size and shape of the skull and the pituitary fossa, to show the changes due to raised intracranial pressure and the presence of fractures. Both left and right lateral projections should be obtained, if possible, when examining a patient with a severe head injury. One of these projections should be taken with the patient in the supine "brow-up" position, to show if intracranial air is present or if there is a fluid level in the sphenoid sinus (see below).

Postero-anterior (PA 20°) projection

The frontal bone, frontal sinus, ethmoidal air-cell system and the orbits are best seen on this projection.

Semi-axial (Towne's) projection

This projection is used to assess the position of the calcified pineal and choroid plexuses, the appearance of the petrous bones, including the internal acoustic meatus and canals, and to show fractures involving the posterior half of the skull.

Submentovertical (basal) projection

This projection is used to demonstrate the basal foramina and fractures involving the skull base.

Arrange to see a standard radiographic examination of the skull being carried out by an experienced radiographer and ask her what she is doing and why. The expertise required to obtain accurate projections of the skull, especially on patients who are unable to cooperate, may surprise you.

What signs do we look for on these projections and what do they mean?

The size and shape of the skull

An assessment of the size and shape of the skull is of particular importance in infants and children. Get used to the concept of craniofacial proportion; that is, a comparison of the size of the cranial and facial structures. It must be said, however, that an x-ray examination of the skull is not the best or cheapest way of finding out if the head is of abnormal size. This is best done by using a tape measure: abnormal skull growth is much easier to detect by serial measurements of head circumference than by radiography. What one can detect radiologically is whether the sutures are abnormally wide and whether the skull is of an abnormal shape.

Assessment of the width of the sutures is difficult in the newborn as the edges of the sutures are rather ill-defined.

Microcephaly (an abnormally small head) can be recognized as the calvarium is invariably abnormally thick, there is absence of the normal convolutional skull markings and the sutures are closed—all signs that the brain is not growing at a normal rate.

The misshapen skull

A shallow posterior fossa, seen on the lateral projection, together with an occipital bone which is concave rather than convex in outline, often occurs in infants with hydrocephalus due to two common developmental abnormalities of the hind brain: cerebellar ectopia and aqueduct stenosis. This deformity may be accompanied by a defect of ossification of the membrane bone of the skull called craniolacuna (Fig. 6.1). This is commonly seen in infants with the more severe forms of spina bifida (meningomyelocoele) which, together with an abnormality of the hind brain, presages the development of hydro-cephalus. Craniolacuna is not due to raised intracranial pressure.

Distinct skull asymmetry in infancy and early childhood is usually of clinical significance. A minor degree of asymmetry is common in children and adults and appears to be unimportant.

Craniostenosis—that is, premature closure of one or more of the cranial sutures—can give rise to severe skull deformity. The sagittal suture is most commonly affected and causes a boat-shaped deformity of the skull (*scapho-cephaly*). Premature stenosis of one of the coronal sutures leads to marked asymmetry of the two halves of the skull (*plagiocephaly*). Another important

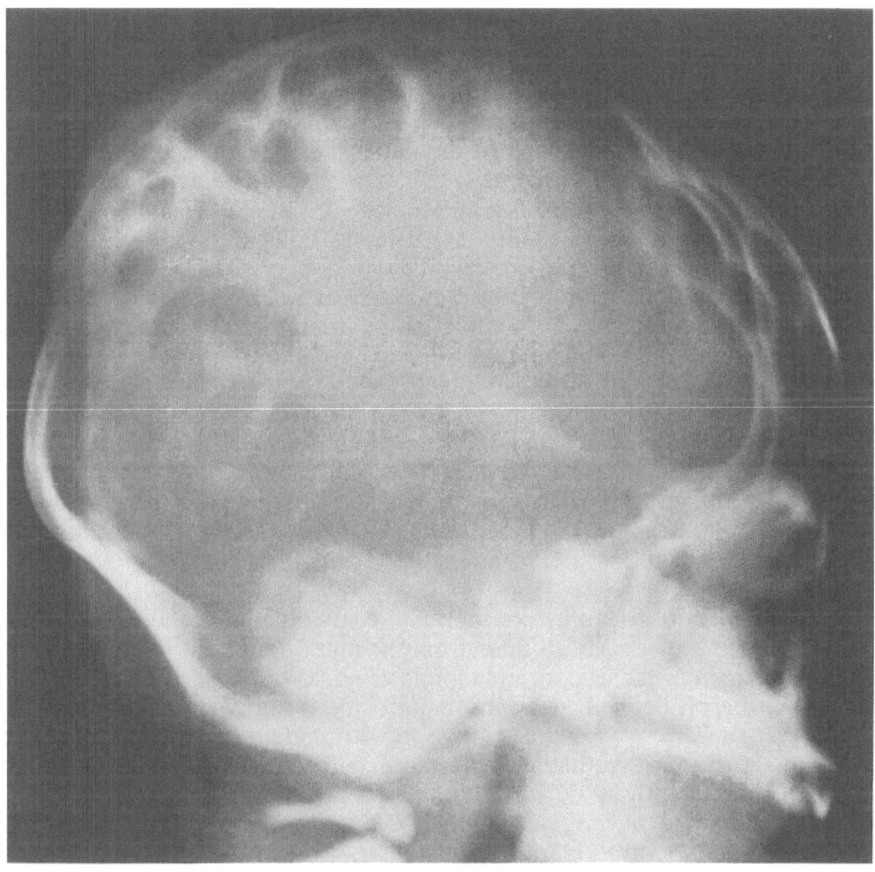

Fig. 6.1. Skull of an infant, lateral projection. There is a defect of ossification of the skull vault (craniolacuna) which is commonly seen in infants with spina bifida (meningomyelocoele). The occipital bone is concave in outline. This is evidence of a developmental abnormality of hind brain. The infant developed hydrocephalus due to aqueduct atresia.

cause of plagiocephaly is underdevelopment of one of the cerebral hemi-spheres, cerebral hypoplasia, due to a prenatal cause or birth trauma. In this condition there is thickening of the calvarium, absence of the normal convolutional markings, and overdevelopment of the frontal sinus and mastoid air-cell system on the affected side. In the Sturge–Weber syndrome (see below) these radiological features are commonly present in addition to visible intracranial calcification.

Another cause of plagiocephaly in children is a juvenile subdural hygroma. This condition, which causes pressure erosion of bone in the anterior part of the middle fossa, and elevation of the lesser wing of sphenoid, is often associated with partial agenesis of the temporal lobe. Neurofibromatosis and arachnoid cysts are other causes of local pressure erosion of bone and skull asymmetry.

Skull fractures

All patients rendered unconscious by a head injury, however briefly, should have an x-ray examination of the skull. This is not for "medico-legal" reasons but to assist in the management of the patient.

The presence of a skull fracture is evidence that the patient has not had a trivial injury, however well he may seem at the time of examination, and should alert you to the possibility that complications may arise. Apart from the relatively rare depressed fracture (which always needs correction), the main purpose of skull films after trauma is to reduce the risk of further damage to the brain from intracranial haemorrhage or a cerebrospinal fluid (CSF) fistula. Most adult patients at risk will have a skull fracture (see below), and for this reason skull radiographs are a useful element in an admission policy for the very large number of patients attending hospital with head injuries each year (about 1 million in the United Kingdom).

A fracture is detectable radiologically in two-thirds of patients who have sustained a severe head injury, and in 30% of the remainder there is clinical evidence of a fracture of the base of the skull. Conversely, the absence of a visible skull fracture does not mean that the patient has not had a severe head injury.

Linear or fissure fractures are the most common skull fractures. It is not usually difficult to distinguish them from the markings on the skull caused by the middle meningeal arteries and diploic veins, as fractures appear "darker" and more sharply defined. A fissure fracture may occur anywhere in the skull. If the fracture line crosses the groove for the middle meningeal artery, be alert to the possibility that an extradural haematoma may be present or develop subsequently. *90% of adult patients with an extradural haematoma have a visible skull fracture, as indeed do 75% of patients with acute intradural (i.e. subdural and intracerebral) haematomas.*

Look for a calcified pineal gland on the semi-axial (Towne's) projection and, if visible, check to see if it is displaced from the midline (see below). If it is, the patient may have an intracranial haematoma and must be admitted immediately and put under continuous observation (Fig. 6.2).

It is a regrettable fact that the morbidity and mortality of acute extradural haematomas are still far too high.

Look to see if the paranasal sinuses and mastoid air-cell systems are normally translucent. If one or more of the sinuses is opaque, look for intracranial air lying over the frontal lobes or above the pituitary fossa, and for a fluid level in the sphenoid sinus on the "brow-up" lateral projection. Intracranial air is unequivocal evidence of a CSF fistula due to a dural tear. A fluid level in the sphenoid sinus (Fig. 6.3) is most commonly due to blood but,

Fig. 6.2. Skull, semi-axial (Towne's) projection. The calcified pineal is displaced 5 mm to the right of midline (*arrow*) due to a left convexity subdural haematoma.

Fig. 6.3. Skull, brow-up lateral projection. No visible fracture in the cranial vault. There is a fluid level (*arrow*) in the sphenoid sinus due to a basal skull fracture with CSF rhinorrhoea.

Fig. 6.2 ▶

Fig. 6.3 ▶

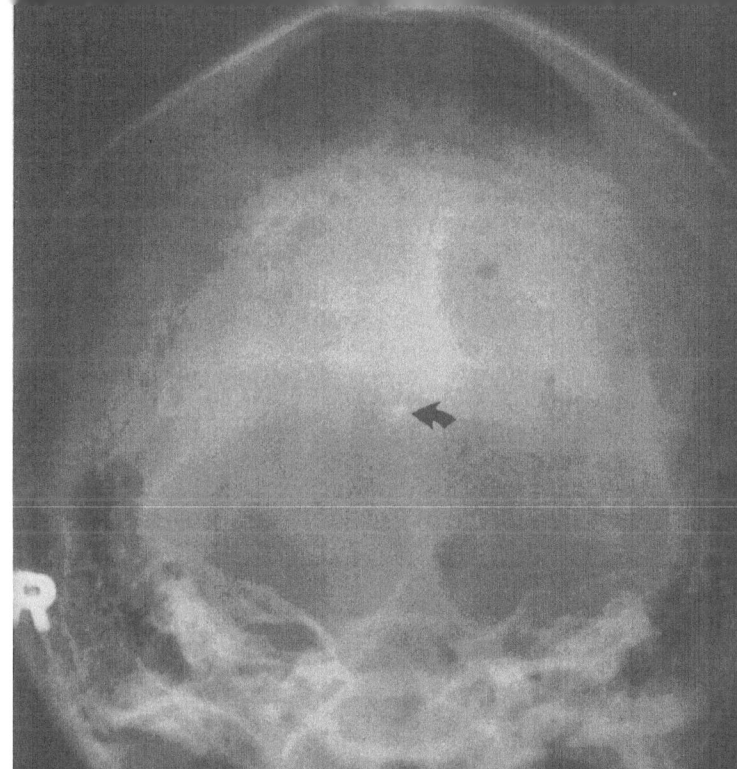

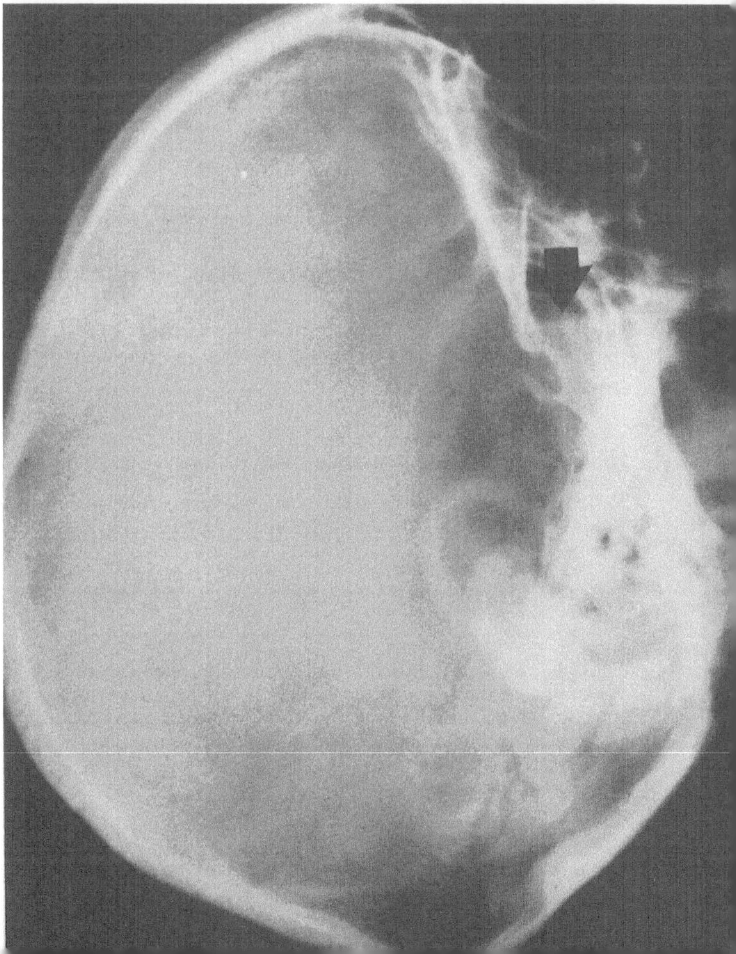

if there is no clinical evidence of an epistaxis, CSF rhinorrhoea is the next most common cause, and this must be excluded by clinical examination. Meningitis commonly occurs if a CSF leak goes undetected and the patient is not put on prophylactic antibiotics.

A serious but less common complication of a dural tear is a collection of air in the brain (pneumocephalus) which acts as a space-occupying lesion and may rupture into the ventricles. This condition may develop days or weeks after the initial head injury.

A comminuted fracture of the skull consists of a number of fissure fractures radiating from the point of impact, which is often depressed. This is sometimes difficult to recognize, especially in children, and it is important to do so as there is some evidence that the incidence of post-traumatic epilepsy is reduced by surgical elevation of the depressed bone. A linear or comminuted fracture with separation of the fragments is said to be diastased. In children some of these diastased fractures progressively enlarge instead of healing. This is due to an associated tear of the underlying dura, with protrusion of the arachnoid which erodes and everts the edges of the fracture by abnormal CSF pulsation. This is called a "growing fracture of childhood".

The cranial sutures may become widened following trauma in children and adults. This traumatic diastasis is due to deformation of the skull at the time of impact, and is one of the hallmarks of a major head injury.

It is possible for a sharp object such as a pencil to penetrate the orbital roof, especially in children. These injuries (which are difficult to demonstrate radiographically) can be overlooked clinically unless one is aware of this possibility. Beware of the "simple" laceration of the upper eyelid in children!

High-velocity penetrating injuries of the skull due to missiles present special diagnostic and management problems which will not be considered here.

Signs of an intracranial space-occupying lesion

An intracranial tumour or other space-occupying lesion can under certain circumstances produce radiological signs which may be detected on standard skull x-rays. These signs include the changes of raised intracranial pressure, displacement of the pineal gland, changes in the overlying bone and intracranial calcification.

Raised intracranial pressure

Raised intracranial pressure is most commonly due to obstructive hydro-cephalus, a space-occupying lesion, or to both of these conditions. Less

-->

Fig. 6.4.a Skull of a child, lateral projection. The sutures are of normal width, as are the convolutional markings of the skull vault. **b** Separation of the coronal suture due to raised intracranial pressure. The increase in the convolutional markings of the skull vault is evidence that the raised intracranial pressure is not of recent origin.

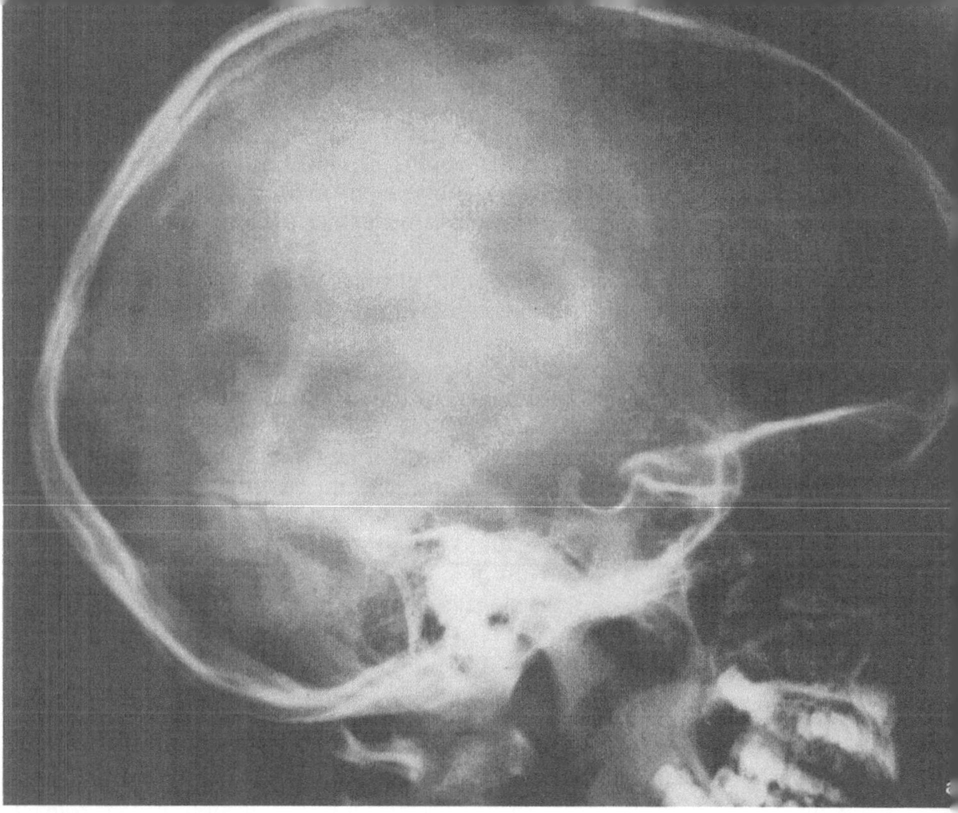

Fig. 6.4.a ▲

Fig. 6.4.b ▼

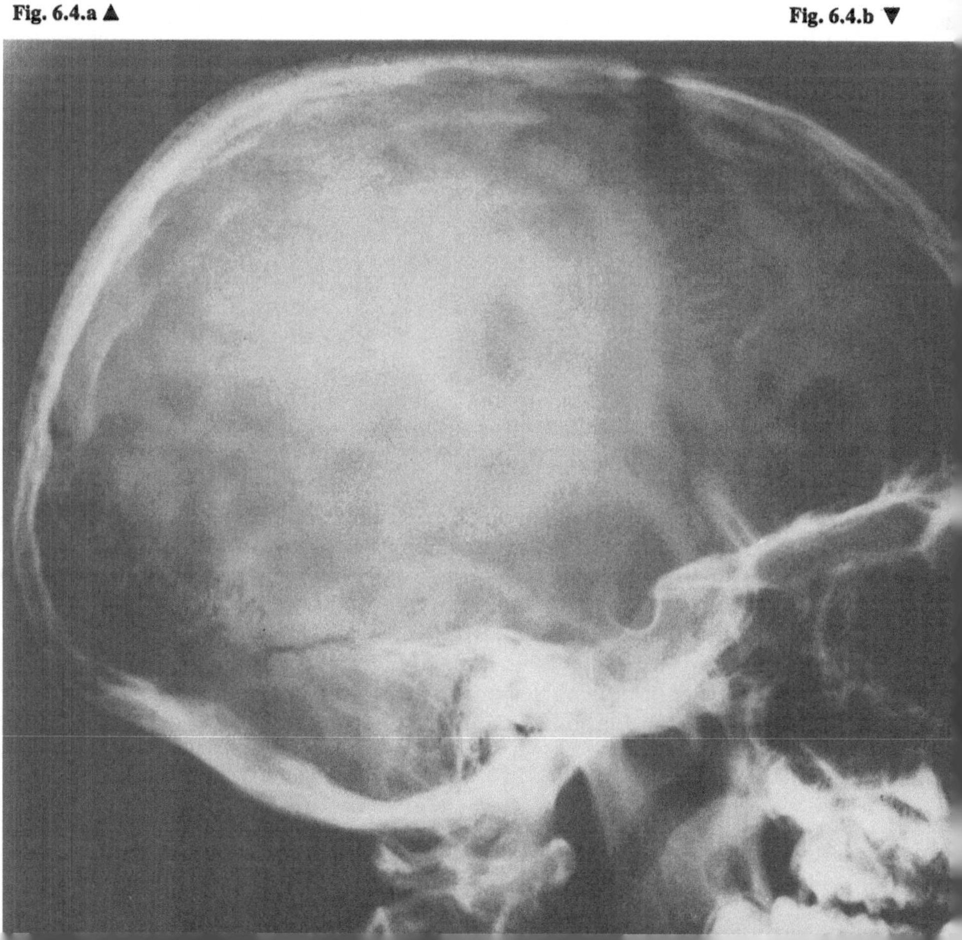

common causes of raised intracranial pressure are benign intracranial hypertension (otitic hydrocephalus and pseudotumour cerebri are the alternative names of this condition), tuberculous meningitis, lead intoxication, a generalized metabolic disorder (e.g. renal failure) and, rarely, certain drugs (corticosteroids and tetracycline).

In children up to about the age of 10 years, a sustained rise in intracranial pressure causes separation of the cranial sutures (Fig. 6.4). This is first seen in the upper part of the coronal sutures and in the sagittal suture, and may appear before there are clinical signs. In patients with long-standing raised intracranial pressure the normal convolutional markings on the inner table of the skull may be exaggerated, giving rise to the so-called 'silverbeaten' appearance. This sign alone is insecure evidence of raised intracranial pressure, as prominent convolutional markings are often seen on the skull x-rays of normal children and young adults. It is a safe rule that a diagnosis of raised intracranial pressure should not be made based solely on the presence of prominent calvarial convolutional markings. After the age of 10 years or thereabouts, suture diastasis does not occur, and the earliest radiological sign of raised intracranial pressure is erosion of the anterior cortex of the dorsum sellae, where it forms the posterior boundary of the pituitary fossa (Fig. 6.5). This change takes several weeks to develop and is normally seen after there is clinical evidence of raised intracranial pressure. Although these changes seem to be confined to the dorsum sellae, they are probably present but less readily visible elsewhere in the skull. Prolonged elevation of intracranial pressure causes erosion of the bony cortex of the floor of the pituitary fossa, which may become enlarged and deepened, and of the anterior fossa, especially the planum sphenoidale and the lesser wings of the sphenoid. These bony changes are thought to be due to abnormal pulsation of CSF, at increased pressure, in the suprasellar cisterns and in dilated third and lateral ventricles.

Space-occupying lesions, wherever they occur, may produce radiological signs of raised intracranial pressure. In patients with a tumour in the posterior fossa, especially children, this may be the only detectable radiological abnormality.

Pineal displacement

A supratentorial space-occupying lesion, be it a tumour or a blood clot, will, unless symmetrically bilateral, displace the midline structures of the brain, including the pineal gland. Calcification of the pineal gland is visible on plain x-rays in about 60% of adults, but is rarely visible in children. This calcification (when visible on a well-positioned semi-axial or Towne's projection) is normally no more than 2 mm from the midline. Accurately measure on this projection the biparietal diameter of the skull from outer table to outer table, at the level of the pineal gland. Halve the measured distance and mark the midpoint on the x-ray film. If the calcified pineal is situated 3 mm or more from the midline, the patient has either a supratentorial space-occupying lesion on one side or an atrophic lesion on the opposite side (see Fig. 6.2).

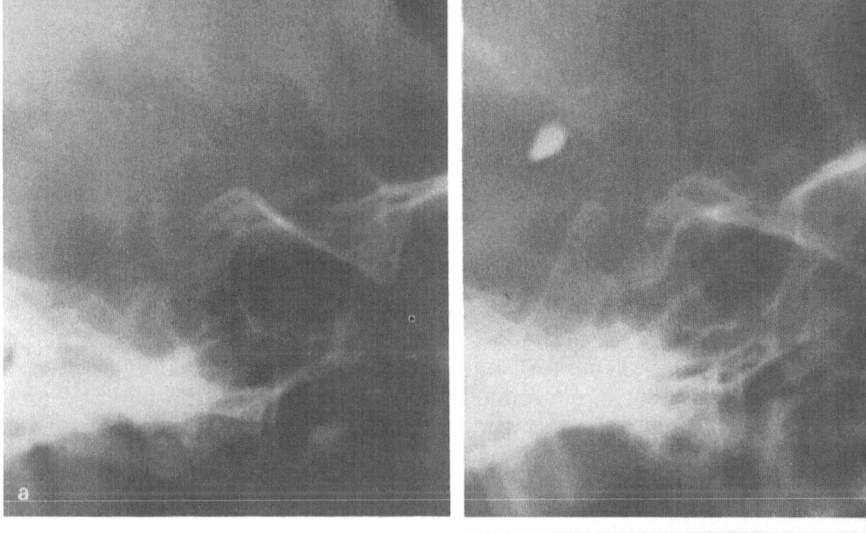

Fig. 6.5, a–c. Adult skull, pituitary fossa, lateral projection. **a** marked reduction in bone density of the dorsum sellae, the floor of the pituitary fossa and to a lesser degree the planum sphenoidale, due to long-standing raised intracranial pressure; **b** same patient: the pressure has been relieved and the bone density is returning to normal; **c** some years later: the pituitary fossa is a little deformed but the bone density is now normal.

Temporal and parietal tumours and haematomas commonly displace the pineal gland from the midline; frontal and occipital lesions do so less frequently. Calcification in the choroid plexus in the region of the trigone of each lateral ventricle is frequently visible on plain films in adults. Although this calcification is not always symmetrical, displacement of one choroid plexus may be seen when there is a space-occupying lesion in the temporal, parietal or occipital regions.

Prominent calvarial vascular grooves

Enlargement and tortuosity of the grooves for the middle meningeal arteries on the inner table of the skull and of the diploic venous channels may be seen in association with a tumour arising from the meninges—a meningioma. This can be a difficult radiological sign to interpret. Look for supporting evidence of enlargement of the foramen spinosum on the basal projection (i.e. the foramen through which the middle meningeal artery enters the skull).

Changes in the overlying bone

Tumours arising from the meninges or the cranial nerves may be associated with changes in the adjacent bone. Meningiomas may cause local overgrowth or erosion of bone, or both. These changes, together with enlarged meningeal grooves, are diagnostic of the presence of an underlying meningioma (Fig. 6.6). A tumour of the optic nerve, commonly a glioma, may produce enlargement of one or both optic canals; a tumour of the eighth nerve, an acoustic neuroma, commonly causes erosion and widening of the adjacent internal acoustic meatus and canal. Tumours arising from other cranial nerves are rare. Primary tumours of the brain rarely produce changes in the overlying bone.

Intracranial calcification

In addition to the calcification in the pineal gland and choroid plexuses visible on plain films, ossification may be seen in the dura, particularly in the walls of the sagittal sinus, in the falx cerebri and in the tentorium cerebelli. In elderly people, dystrophic calcification is commonly seen in the carotid arteries on either side of the pituitary fossa. Some primary tumours of the brain calcify

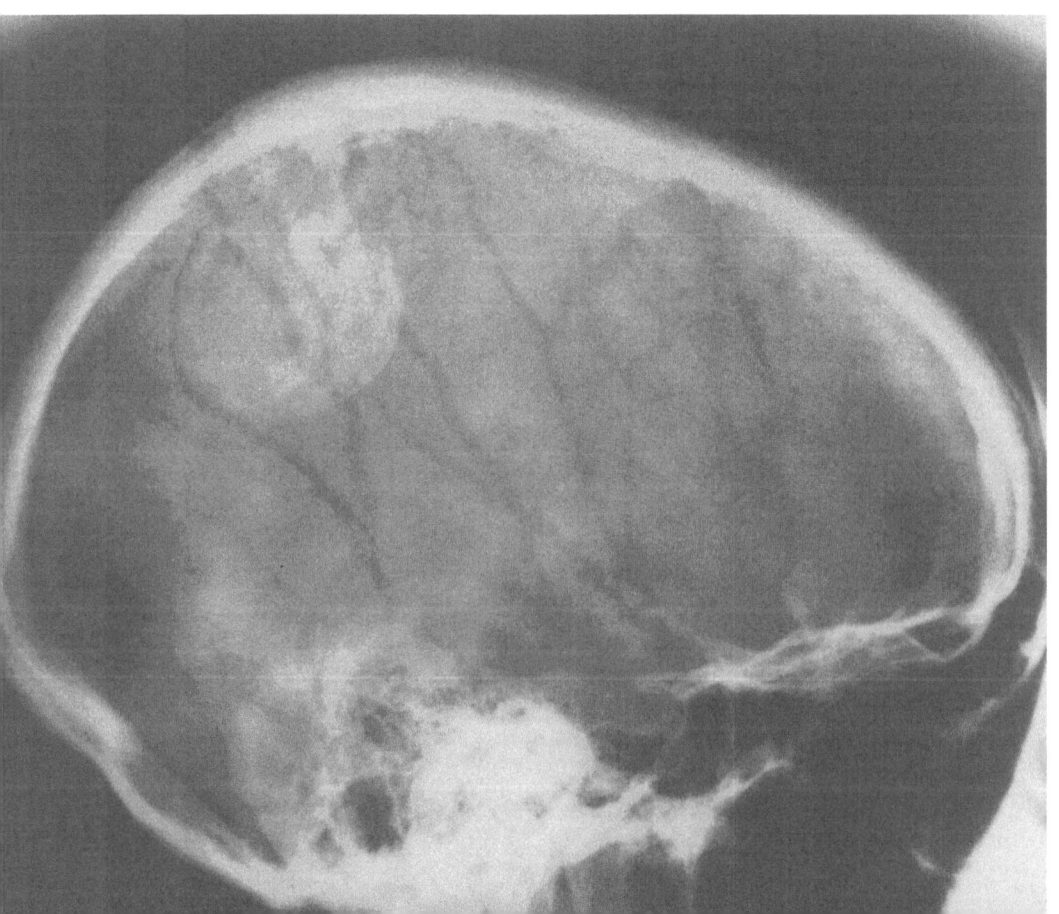

sufficiently for this to be detectable by plain radiography. Cranio-pharyngiomas, tumours which arise in Rathké's pouch, commonly calcify in both children and adults. The calcification, which is situated above or in the pituitary fossa, is seen in about 60% of patients.

Oligodendrogliomas may also be calcified sufficiently for them to be detectable on plain films, as are a small percentage of low-grade astro-cytomas. The rare pinealoma which normally presents in childhood is commonly visible due to calcification within it. Some extracerebral tumours show visible calcification, particularly chordomas, which arise in notochordal remnants within the skull. Calcification is occasionally seen in meningiomas but this is less common than, and may be confused with, hyperostosis of the overlying bone.

Calcification is commonly seen in the walls of giant partly thrombosed intracranial aneurysms in adults and is occasionally, although rarely, visible in the walls of the abnormal vessels of cerebral arteriovenous malformation. Parallel lines of calcification in the posterior parietal and occipital regions of one cerebral hemisphere conforming to the convolutions of the cerebral gyri, when found in association with a naevus in the cutaneous distribution of the trigeminal nerve, is the hallmark of encephalotrigeminal angiomatosis (the Sturge–Weber syndrome).

The pituitary fossa

The appearance of the normal pituitary fossa varies quite widely from individual to individual. There is a fairly close fit between the size of the pituitary gland and the fossa in most individuals; it follows that enlargement of the gland will usually produce pressure erosion of the surrounding bone and an increase in size of the fossa.

The commonest pituitary tumour in adults is the chromophobe adenoma, which usually presents with symptoms of hypopituitarism and chiasmal compression. This tumour invariably causes enlargement of the pituitary fossa, which is detectable radiographically (Fig. 6.7).

About 80% of pituitary tumours which are associated with elevated growth-hormone levels and cause gigantism or acromegaly have radiological evidence of enlargement of the pituitary fossa. Few patients with Cushing's syndrome have this radiological evidence. After bilateral adrenalectomy, however, a rapid increase in size of a basophil tumour of the pituitary may cause sellar enlargement as part of Nelson's syndrome. Patients with hyperprolactinaemia due to a microadenoma of the pituitary gland rarely have plain-film evidence of enlargement of the pituitary fossa.

Fig. 6.6. Adult skull, lateral projection. Reduction in bone density of the dorsum sellae due to raised intracranial pressure. Enlargement of the calvarial, meningeal and dural vascular channels associated with a calcified meningioma in the parietal region. (Visible calcification in menin-giomas is not very common.)

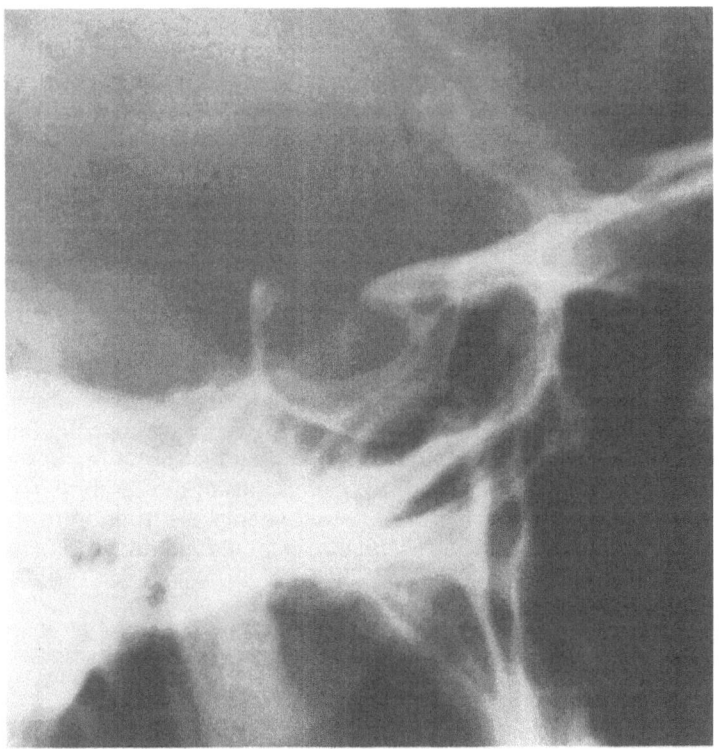

Fig. 6.7. Adult skull. Pituitary fossa, lateral projection. Asymmetric enlargement of the pituitary fossa due to a pituitary tumour. Chromophobe adenoma.

A craniopharyngioma, chiasmal glioma, a dilated third ventricle, extension of the subarachnoid space into the sella (the empty sella syndrome), a cavernous carotid aneurysm and tumours of the sphenoid sinus may all produce changes in the sella which can be difficult to distinguish from those due to a pituitary tumour.

The skull as a bone

The skull is affected by many of the conditions that involve the rest of the skeleton. Paget's disease can cause gross skull deformity due to bone thickening, and basilar invagination due to bone softening. Both the skull and facial structures may be affected by fibrous dysplasia. The skull is a common site for bony metastases. Carcinomas of the breast and bronchus are the commonest primary tumours which give rise to osteolytic metastases in the calvarium. Sclerotic metastases from a primary prostatic carcinoma usually affect the skull base.

84

X-rays of the skull are commonly requested on patients with multiple myelomatosis as the frequency of involvement of the skull and the radiological appearances are considered to be of diagnostic importance. The skull is affected in many of the bone dysplasias, for example achondroplasia, cleidocranial dysostosis and osteogenesis imperfecta. Changes may be seen in the skull in metabolic bone disease, in the haemoglobinopathies (thalassaemia and sickle-cell anaemia) and in the histiocytic diseases (eosinophilic granuloma).

Special problems in the elderly

The bone density of the skull often looks abnormal in elderly people. This is usually due to a combination of a reduction of total bone content and the osteoporosis which is commonly present in post-menopausal women. The reduced density of the dorsum sellae due to these conditions may mimic that due to raised intracranial pressure. Systemic arterial hypertension, which is not uncommon in the elderly, may also produce similar appearances.

The skulls of middle-aged and elderly women frequently show an endosteal nodular thickening of the frontal bone, sparing only the midline groove for the superior sagittal sinus. This so-called hyperostosis frontalis interna (HFI) is without clinical significance. Thinning of the outer table of the parietal bones may be seen in elderly people of both sexes and is of no clinical importance.

Old people who are confused fall out of bed and those who fall out of bed often become confused. An x-ray examination is commonly requested to "exclude a skull fracture", which is rarely, if ever, present. The examination, however, is not without value as elderly people can develop a chronic subdural haematoma after a relatively trivial head injury. Examine the skull films carefully and note the position of the calcified pineal on the semi-axial (Towne's) projection. If it is midline all is well for the time being. If the patient remains confused, repeat the skull x-ray examination in 1 to 2 weeks and if the pineal remains central in position, a surgically significant subdural haematoma can be excluded with confidence.

Parting shot

Radiology plays an important part in the diagnosis and management of patients with suspected intracranial disease. X-rays of the skull and chest are essential before proceeding to more expensive (cranial computed tomography) or invasive (cerebral angiography) neuroradiological investigations. If we ignore this rule, we imperil our patients and our reputations.

7.   About Learning to See and Think

The presence of a chapter on such a nebulous topic may seem an intrusion in a book devoted to radiology—of all medical disciplines, that most deeply indebted for its origins to physics, and still intimately dependent for its continuous development on the technology of light, heat and sound. I shall add to the shock by introducing my theme with somewhat allegorical talk, hoping to turn your thoughts into unaccustomed grooves. But be patient; allegories (pictures in which meaning is symbolically represented) are no strangers to radiology. The raw data of this subject are pictures, images; and you may be working with several different kinds of images of the same thing. You will need to learn their codes: not only how they were made, so that you can recognize what they represent anatomically, but what they mean (allegorically), what inferences they can help you to make about the patient's health or sickness.

If, encouraged that way by preclinical "basic science" courses, you still seek diamond-hard precision and clarity of things seen in unchanging one-to-one relationships, simple and straightforward, recall that clinical medicine presents a different face. Diamonds and graphite are at atomic level the same substance and, standardized for weight, would appear the same in a radiograph. It is because the atoms are differently related to each other that to ordinary senses one seems hard, clear and colourless as pure water, and the other soft and blacker than night.

Recall that still more complicated kinds of relationships confound bio-logical matters, including those concerning the ways students learn, and doctors treat their patients. A person contains a sample of most of the atoms present in this planet, compounded into molecules of mind-boggling variety. Within this body different organs, in orderly arrangement, are separated by selectively permeable barriers; they interact with each other in complicated but orderly fashions. Within each organ there are different cells and extracellular components; within each cell different organelles—the closer you look the more you see. Now lift your eyes from the microscope; consider that each person is an individual, definable as persisting in time and space but, like a cell, he is an open system selectively permeable to the environment, in its mental as well as physical aspects. Psychologically, the most important parts of his environment are other people, and in attempting to diagnose and treat an individual the doctor needs to look also at another level of organization—at his family, his work site and so on. For sure, the greatest threats to health and sanity come at the still more complicated sociological level of clashes between economic or religious classes, or between nations.

We must keep these complexities of interaction in mind when considering learning. The jug-and-bottle concept, of the student as a passive empty receptacle into which the teacher pours knowledge, is oversimple, but still affects our educational arrangements: they are caricatured in the picture of a mediaeval school room (Fig. 7.1). The teacher's authority over the pupils is tacitly emphasized in various ways—he is not only bigger than them, but sits on a higher seat, and wears a tall hat; his book is bigger than theirs; he faces one way, and they the other; he is separated from them by the lectern. He holds a birch for beating them, and his assistant is ready to ridicule them with a donkey's head when they are stupid.

Compare this social milieu with that of another picture, Rembrandt's sketch of two women helping a toddler to learn to walk (Fig. 7.2). They have put a padded hat on his head in case he falls, they hold his hands, bending their heads towards him. One points the way with outstretched arm, gesturing into his future, of conditions she will never see, cannot imagine.

The mediaeval classroom is a set-up designed to ensure that what the teacher gives, and what the pupils are expected to swallow, is dogma to be absorbed as such, unquestioned now, and unchanged for years to come. In our times of rapid technological change, even if the student can take in all the "teacher's" knowledge, much of it will be out of date by the time he needs it

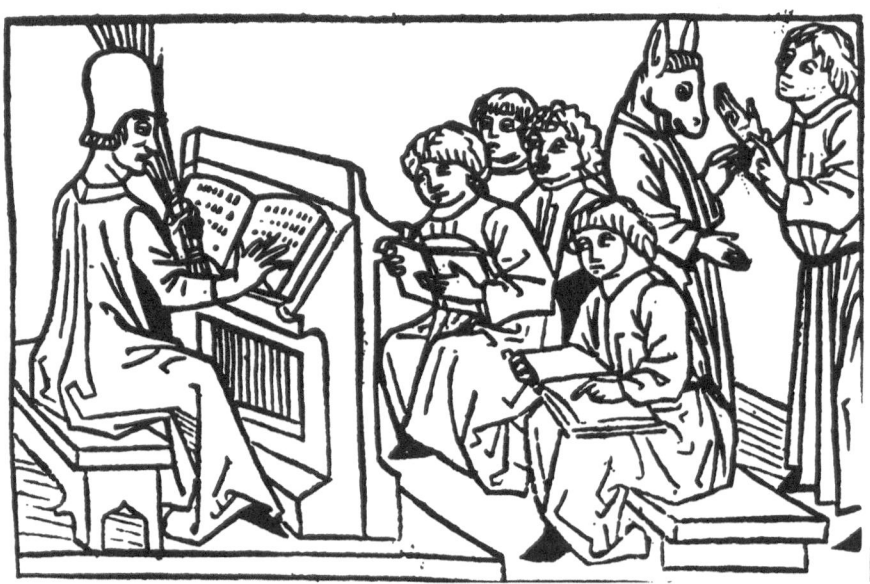

Fig. 7.1. "A schoolroom". Rodericus Zamorensis, c.1475. (By courtesy of Trustees of the British Museum)

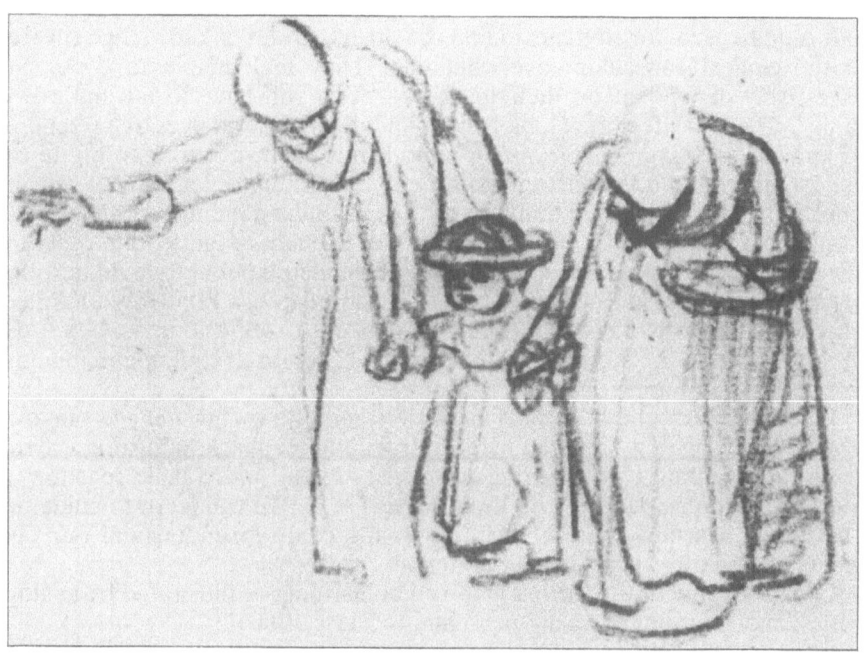

Fig. 7.2. "Two women teaching a child to walk". Rembrandt, 1640. (By courtesy of Trustees of the British Museum)

for use in medical practice. Moreover, the pupil is not a passive, empty receptacle into which the teacher pours knowledge, but always has to undertake considerable work to rearrange the contents of his mind to accommodate new material. And the difficulties are in detail idiosyncratic and not easily understood by either teacher or pupil. A quotation from Laing's (1970) "Knots" expresses the difficulties of communication and understanding:

> I don't know *what* it is I don't know
>   and yet am supposed to know.
> and I feel I look stupid
>   if I seem both not to know it
>   and not to know *what* it is I don't know.
> Therefore I pretend I know it.
>   This is nerve-racking
>   since I don't know what I must pretend to know.
> Therefore I pretend to know everything...
>
> You may know what I don't know, but not
>   that I don't know it,
> and I can't tell you. So you will have to tell me everything.

It is quite usual for students to find the sheer amount of knowledge covered in the clinical curriculum overwhelming. They feel unable to cope, and excessively dependent on their teachers—"You will have to tell me everything". They may feel they look stupid, and defend themselves by pretending to know everything. This frame of mind is not conducive to learning to see and to think, and it is quite antagonistic to enjoyment of learning to see and think. The answer lies, we think, in each of us understanding more about our own behaviour. A wag has described the human brain as the best and cheapest general computer assembled by unskilled labour. I would add that even the cleverest and wisest of us use much of it in a relatively unskilled, unsophisticated way; and that each person needs to learn to make better use of his brain, to be able to exploit his own cerebral equipment in more productive and happier ways.

We are only at the beginning of understanding how to manage our own brains. Working in groups can help by providing feedback: adjusting ways of seeing and thinking by comparing and contrasting the individual's reactions to the same stimulus pattern with those of his peers. We can learn to guide our own future learning more efficiently, having come to understand our own habits of thinking and behaving better.

Consider some of the factors involved in learning, as illustrated by analogy with demonstrations of visual perception. These show:

1) That the uptake of information is highly selective and interpretative, and
2) That we are mostly quite unaware of how our judgements, about what it is that we are looking at, are made.

Two groups of factors which affect the uptake of information can be usefully considered: those of the individual's past experience and those of the context in which the information is received. Discussion in a small group brings to light great individual variability in responses to the same information. Each person is necessarily egocentric in his perceptions. By comparison and contrast of his own judgement with those of other members of the group, each can become aware, as he previously was not, of the factors that most powerfully affected his own interpretations. When these are brought into consciousness they can be subjected to evaluation by himself and other members of the group.

Interaction in small groups can serve another important function: teamwork. The practice of medicine now depends on experts working together to get information one from the other. Taking a clinical history is one, perhaps unexpected, example. You are learning to get information from the patient who is an expert on his own history—in some aspects of it *the* expert. Later you will need to get information from various other experts about the observations and tests they have made on your patient. Sometimes their investigations have been done independently of the clinician, who merely asks for certain data and receives the specialist's report. Sometimes, indeed, the specialist is supposed to be more objective if he works blindly, not knowing the patient or the case history, and bringing an "innocent eye" to the investigation. But any radiologist will tell of gross errors he has made when not sufficiently informed about the patient.

These pages have put forward a different relationship between the patient, clinical medicine and radiology. With the increasing range of highly specific techniques, it makes more sense for the expert to be in the picture *before* the question is specified, i.e. for radiologists not only to answer a question but to collaborate with the clinician in posing it. We are concerned not only with the *transmission* of information, with all the problems of communication that that involves—goodness knows, complicated enough. We are trying, in collaboration with clinicians, to formulate more precisely the questions that should be asked so that the actual *eliciting* of information becomes a joint effort. The ability to do this economically and effectively involves skills in human relationships.

Some believe that people are born with or without such skills, but I think that quite a lot can be done to cultivate them, though at present our main methods of educating people, inspired by the jug-and-bottle idea, are not very helpful. Many students are inhibited from asking questions when invited to do so after a lecture. They are terrified of admitting ignorance or stupidity or making fools of themselves in public. Behaving passively, they do not feel that it is part of their job to help the teacher to teach, nor do they recognize that it is likely that other students would like to know the answer to the question, but maybe have been unable to formulate it for themselves, let alone voice it in the lecture theatre. Such ways of perceiving one's relation to a source of knowledge will be as unhelpful to the doctor as they are to the student, but collaborative work can help to dissolve the difficulties, and help to establish constructive self-confidence as a sound basis for new adventures. Away with the birch and the donkey's head: we can provide the crash helmet and a steadying hand for each other.

Reference

Laing RD (1970) Knots. Tavistock, London, p 56

Subject Index